Controversies in C

David W. Haslam • Arya M. Sharma
Carel W. le Roux
Editors

Controversies in Obesity

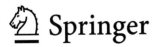 Springer

Editors
David W. Haslam
Watton Place Clinic
Watton-at-Stone
Hertfordshire
UK

Arya M. Sharma
Department of Medicine
University of Alberta
Edmonton
Alberta
Canada

Carel W. le Roux
Department of Pathology
Diabetes Complications
Research Centre
University College Dublin
Dublin
Ireland

ISBN 978-1-4471-2833-5   ISBN 978-1-4471-2834-2   (eBook)
DOI 10.1007/978-1-4471-2834-2
Springer London Heidelberg New York Dordrecht

Library of Congress Control Number: 2013956425

Printed on acid-free paper

Springer is part of Springer Science+Business Media (www.springer.com)

Foreword

The Confusions and Controversies Associated with Obesity

For those of us who have been involved in the obesity story in modern times it is always frustrating that there is so much confusion, debate, and misunderstanding relating to the subject. As scientists it was difficult for us to be considered as involved in any challenging, let alone important and significant, research. Everybody seemed to have an opinion based on their own experience and interpretation, and even highly trained doctors seemed to rely on what they picked up in passing from newspapers or women's magazines to condition their views. It is therefore not surprising that some of these features exist more than 40 years later after a huge amount of work has opened up a wide range of issues. Now we are more than ever confronted with different views in medical practice and in assessing the dietary and other factors responsible for weight gain and its complications. This is before we even begin to consider the array of approaches to treatment and the seemingly bewildering challenge of prevention with ideas ranging from education to school management, the value of gymnastic facilities, private slimming clinics, urban planning and traffic policies, and even fiscal and legislative measures.

We should not be intimidated by all these issues but recognize that it is a wonderful sign that the topic is now considered so important that it involves everybody from basic scientists to physiologists, endocrinologists, neuroscientists, and psychologists as well as the medical profession in an array of specialists. Public health specialists are also now locked into health economics and policy making as they assess the parallels with combating tobacco and alcohol use.

This book deals with a whole range of issues where there is so much uncertainty, but it is a natural part of the process of gaining an ever-increasing understanding of the multiple forms of obesity and how to not only understand the underlying mechanisms involved in their manifestation but also discriminate the most suitable forms of treatment and prevention of a condition that is now taking central stage in places such as the United Nations General Assembly and the Treasuries of the world as the predictions of an unsustainable economic health burden emerge across the world.

W. Philip T. James
International Association for the Study of Obesity,
Charles Darwin House
London, UK

Contents

Contributors

Kristine H. Allin Faculty of Health and Medical Sciences, The Novo Nordisk Foundation Center for Basic Metabolic Research, Section of Metabolic Genetics, University of Copenhagen, Copenhagen, Denmark

Richard L. Atkinson Obetech Obesity Research Center, Obetech, LLC, Richmond, VA, USA

Matthew S. Capehorn Rotherham Institute for Obesity (RIO), Clifton Medical Centre, Rotherham, South Yorkshire, UK

Shamil A. Chandaria National Obesity Forum, London, UK

Rajesh Chauhan Watton Place Clinic, Watton at Stone, Hertfordshire, UK

Debbie R.J. Cook Center for Health and Human Performance, London, UK

Melanie J. Davies Diabetes Research Unit, College of Medicine, Biological Sciences and Psychology, University of Leicester, Leicester Diabetes Centre, Leicester General Hospital, Leicester, Leicestershire, UK

Bertrand R. de Silva Novasom Inc, Glen Burnie, MD, USA

Jean-Pierre Despres Québec Heart and Lung Institute, Québec City, QC, Canada

Nikhil V. Dhurandhar Infections and Obesity Lab, Pennington Biomedical Research Center, Louisiana State University System, Baton Rouge, LA, USA

John B. Dixon Primary Care Research Unit, Clinical Obesity Research, and Weight Assessment and Management Clinic, Baker IDI Heart and Diabetes Institute, Monash University, Melbourne, VIC, Australia

Damian Edwards Department of Behavioural Interventions, National Obesity Forum, London, UK

Paul J. Gately Carnegie Faculty of Sport and Education, Leeds Metropolitan University, Leeds, West Yorkshire, UK

Laura J. Gray Department of Health Sciences, University of Leicester, Leicester, Leicestershire, UK

Julian Paul Hamilton-Shield Biomedical Research Unit in Nutrition and Bristol, Royal Hospital for Children, University of Bristol, Bristol, UK

David W. Haslam Doctor's Surgery, Watton Place Clinic, Watton at Stone, UK

Susan A. Jebb Human Nutrition Research, Medical Research Council, Cambridge, UK

Kamlesh Khunti Diabetes Research Unit, University of Leicester, Leicester, UK

Abdul Fattah Lakhdar Department of Diabetes and Endocrinology, Barts Health NHS Trust, Whipps Cross University Hospital, Leytonstone, London, UK

Michael E.J. Lean School of Medicine, MVLS, Human Nutrition, University of Glasgow, Glasgow, UK

Wen Bun Leong Diabetes and Endocrinology,
Birmingham Heartlands Hospital,
Heart of England NHS Foundation Trust,
Birmingham, West Midlands, UK

Carel W. le Roux Department of Pathology, Diabetes
Complications Research Centre, Conway Institute,
University College Dublin, Dublin, Ireland

Terry Maguire, School of Pharmacy, Queen's University
of Belfast, Belfast, Antrim, Northern Ireland, UK

Aseem Malhotra Department of Cardiology,
Royal Free University Hospital, London, UK

Oluf Pedersen Faculty of Health and Medical Sciences,
The Novo Nordisk Foundation Center for Basic Metabolic
Research, Section of Metabolic Genetics, University
of Copenhagen, Copenhagen, Denmark

Kirsi H. Pietiläinen Obesity Research Unit, Biomedicum
Helsinki, University of Helsinki and Central Hospital,
Helsinki, Finland

Henry J. Purcell Department of Cardiology, Royal
Brompton Hospital, London, UK

Neville J. Rigby International Obesity Forum, London, UK

Stephan Rössner Apple Bay Obesity Research Centre,
Bromma, Sweden

Arya M. Sharma Department of Medicine,
University of Alberta, Edmonton, AB, Canada

Boyd A. Swinburn Section of Epidermiology and
Biostatistics, School of Population Health, University
of Auckland, Auckland, New Zealand

Shahrad Taheri Department of Endocrinology,
School of Clinical and Experimental Medicine,
University of Birmingham, Birmingham, Edgbaston,
West Midlands, UK

Fred Turok Department of Health, Responsibility Deal
Physical Activity Network, London, UK

Tim S. Waters The Hip and Knee Unit, West Hertfordshire
Hospitals NHS Trust, Watford, Hertfordshire, UK

Paul A. Whaley Cancer Prevention and Education Society,
Axminster, Devon, UK

Dennis Wiedman Department of Global and Sociocultural
Studies, School of International and Public Affairs, SIPA
327, Florida International University, Miami, FL, USA

Gary Wittert Discipline of Medicine,
University of Adelaide, Adelaide, SA, Australia

Part I
Introduction

Chapter 1
Obesity: Why Bother?

Stephan Rössner

Over the last 20 years or so, most clinical papers on obesity and obesity-related matters have started in more or less the same way:

- Obesity is a global epidemic. WHO prevalence data are continuously referenced [1].
- The consequences of this explosion can be extrapolated with horrifying prevalence data to be anticipated in a near future. Although a reduced incidence may possibly have been seen, there have never been so many obese individuals on earth as today.
- More people on earth now die of overnutrition rather than undernutrition.
- Obesity is closely related to a number of comorbidities, type 2 diabetes generally coming first, but more and more diseases affecting practically every organ system have been found to be associated.
- Our genes remain essentially unchanged, whereas the environment has been dramatically altered during the last decades.

S. Rössner, MD, PhD
Apple Bay Obesity Research Centre,
Snackparken 7, Bromma S-16753, Sweden
e-mail: stephan@rossner.se

D.W. Haslam et al. (eds.), *Controversies in Obesity*,
DOI 10.1007/978-1-4471-2834-2_1,
© Springer-Verlag London 2014

- Physical activity demands become smaller and smaller with mechanization.
- The food industry is responsible for having created a "toxic" environment.

These facts are constantly reiterated but have become so trivial that it seems a waste of space and paper to ruminate them. We know about them, and did so several decades ago, and so the crucial question remains: Why has so little happened?

In 2011, several papers were published in the Lancet coming from a well-known group of international experts, led by Boyd Swinburn [2–5]. Although this represents a valuable summary of the present situation, the key messages are well known to each and everybody, not only the experts but often also to policymakers and, in many cases, also to the public. The authors state [2] that the global food system promotes obesity in various different ways; mechanization reduces our energy expenditure; individuals are not to blame because they respond predictably to this so-called toxic environment, but governments have generally given in, indicating that body weight control is an individual responsibility.

In almost every modern society, nobody wants to be fat today. Studies suggest that unfortunate obese subjects might be willing to give an arm, or 10 years of their lives, could they only master their weight problems. The strong forces, governed by our Stone Age genes, which once were essential for survival, now wreck our chances to adjust food intake, once food technology has been refined to deliver highly palatable dishes we simply cannot resist. A commonly asked question is why people are obese, despite knowing these basic facts. An equally relevant question may be why there are any lean people left at all.

In many countries activities now begin to take place. For example, in a comment to the four Lancet papers, Dietz summarizes some creative US initiatives with focus both on children and adults [6]. Still that pace is not enough, and when programs are initiated, proper evaluation, rather than wishful thinking, is of outmost importance. Highly educated decision makers see obesity, a stigma of the lower socioeconomic classes, as gluttony, sloppiness, and lack of will power and are hence unwilling to act. There are exceptions. The Netherlands (ironically with one of the lower obesity prevalence rates in Europe) is an example of a society in which an integrated approach has been developed [7].

One of the main problems is that obesity is such a multifaceted condition that no single approach will be sufficient. To eradicate an infectious disease, caused by a known vector, is a monofocal task. For some behaviors, abstinence is the rule (smoking, alcohol, drugs), but we need to eat a few times every day, and, hence, the problem is to develop strategies that allow the victims of obesity to maintain a weight-controlling lifestyle with which they can comply continuously.

To prevent and treat obesity affects so many different parts of our society. Prevention of obesity starts with pregnant mothers, requires support from early childhood onwards into adult life, needs restructuring of our physical environment to promote activity, and requires novel approaches to the whole food delivery system and the adaptation of new behaviors, where media can help. Legislation in various ways is thought by many to be the only way to achieve some of these targets.

Obesity is associated with an increased mortality but is a slow killer, and a politician supporting any kind of program will generally not see the effects during the time of his or her political career. For someone whose horizon is the next election 4 years ahead, investing in the promotion of anti-obesity projects is no priority. Other chronic conditions are different. With dialysis a patient with severe uremia may live reasonably well for a number of years, but if treatment is withheld, the patient is dead within a fortnight. To withhold strategies to prevent and treat obesity results in no obvious and immediate such consequences.

When ministries responsible for the health and welfare of their people have generally failed to act responsibly, help may come from elsewhere. An interesting example comes from the Swedish Ministry of Finance, which set down a working party to analyze the costs of obesity to society [8]. That obesity is costly in many different ways is already well known, but this systematic update of the direct and indirect costs of obesity in a country that is still less plagued by obesity than most others in Europe and elsewhere may send an important signal to politicians to get their act together. For example, production loss because of overweight + obesity in a country of 9.3 million inhabitants amounts to €1.6 billion/year with a rise between 40 and 80 % by the year 2020.

In the USA, severe childhood obesity is now becoming so prevalent that the ensuing type 2 diabetes surfaces already during puberty. It does not require much calculating skill to realize that when these young people reach early middle age, many of them will have worn out their kidneys as a consequence of their diabetes and be ready for dialysis (and, if possible, and for a minority, transplantation), involving huge long-term costs to society and the individual. Scientists in the obesity field have been rightly frustrated.

Prevalence data about the explosion have not impressed enough. Possibly the ensuing dramatic financial consequences may send a stronger signal. And, however cynical it may sound, the depressing outcome in the severely obese child of a top politician may have a stronger impetus than any scientific data.

References

1. WHO. Global strategy on diet, physical activity and health. Geneva: World Health Organization; 2004. http://www.who.int/dietphysicalactivity/en/.
2. Swinburn BA, Sacks G, Hall KD, McPherson K, Finegood DT, Moodie ML, et al. The global obesity pandemic: shaped by global drivers and local environments. Lancet. 2011;378:804–14.
3. Wang YC, McPherson K, Marsh T, Gortmaker SL, Brown M. Health and economic burden of the projected obesity trends in the USA and the UK. Lancet. 2011;378:815–25.
4. Hall KD, Sacks G, Chandramohan D, Chow CC, Wang YC, Gortmaker SL, et al. Quantification of the effect of energy imbalance on bodyweight. Lancet. 2011;378:826–37.

5. Gortmaker SL, Swinburn BA, Levy D, Carter R, Mabry PL, Finegood DT, et al. Changing the future of obesity: science, policy, and action. Lancet. 2011;378:838–47.
6. Dietz WH. Reversing the tide of obesity. Lancet. 2011;378:744–5.
7. Renders CM, Halberstadt J, Frenkel CS, Rosenmöller P, Seidell JC, Hirasing RA. Tackling the problem of overweight and obesity: the Dutch approach. Obes Facts. 2010;3(4):267–72.
8. Rössner S. What ministry takes obesity seriously? Obes Facts. 2011;4:339–40.

Part II
Sociopolitical

Chapter 2
Too Late to Challenge the Modern Obesity Epidemic?

Neville J. Rigby

The origins of obesity reside in the complexity of human genetics and metabolism interacting with variable exogenous factors. These external influences range from food availability and physical activity to less tangible influences, such as in utero conditioning and epigenetic effects, and even potentially to endocrine disrupting chemicals in the environment. The over-played popular message is that obesity merely relates to an energy in/energy out equation and that people who gain weight merely eat too much but do too little. This has been promulgated especially as the mantra of the global food and beverage industries, diverting attention from their efforts to seek ever-increasing consumption of their products. The mantra ignores the complexity of the issue and is misused to shift the "blame" for obesity to individuals, who we are told need to be "educated" to make the right "personal lifestyle choices."

It is also a convenient assumption that early man and woman were so active hunting and gathering, enjoying the resulting Stone Age diet, that they had little chance to become fat. Indeed it may well be the case, as Boyd Eaton has argued, that much of present-day noncommunicable disease, including obesity, is due to our having turned away from the

N.J. Rigby
International Obesity Forum,
C/o 4 Moreton Place, London SW1V 2NP, UK
e-mail: nevillerigby@aol.com

D.W. Haslam et al. (eds.), *Controversies in Obesity*,
DOI 10.1007/978-1-4471-2834-2_2,
© Springer-Verlag London 2014

ancestral diets to which we remain genetically attuned [1]. But an examination of Upper Paleolithic "Venuses," tiny artifacts representing the earliest sculptures of and by Homo sapiens, suggests that obesity was certainly evident, despite the primitive diet, even if the prevalence cannot be conjectured at despite the high predominance of obesity among these figurines [2]. The most recent discovery of the Hohle Fels Venus pushed back the clock on these early depictions of obesity to 35,000 years ago – 5–10 millennia earlier than the Venus of Willendorf, a maquette replica of which is awarded every 4 years to a prominent scientist for their distinguished contribution to obesity research [3].

If people in the Stone Age apparently witnessed, and perhaps even revered, obesity, they can hardly be charged with failing to make the correct "lifestyle choices"; surely it follows that the human race is now at even greater risk in the present-day "toxic" environment, which leaves us very few requirements and opportunities for worthwhile physical activity, and, as Boyd Eaton has pointed out, replaces a natural diet with an industrialized food supply combining an abundance of fats and sugar unavailable in the past. How much greater must the risk of developing obesity now be?

The answer should be clear to everyone. We have witnessed in a little over three decades the growth of the modern obesity epidemic. Obesity prevalence is no longer measured in tiny percentages. More than one-third of US and Mexican adults is obese, more than one-quarter of adults too in the UK, Australia, and New Zealand [4]. Across OECD countries, one in five children is overweight or obese. However, many countries still rely on flawed self-reported surveys that underestimate the prevalence, while Asian countries are advised to lower the bar to obtain a realistic assessment of the scale of their problem. Although the WHO standard cutoff point of BMI $\geq$30 provides a generalized benchmark, it fails to reflect the diffuse spectrum encompassed by obesity and its concomitant health risks. Thus, a WHO estimate of overweight and obesity in China of nearly 22 % contrasts with China's own Working Group on Obesity estimate of 28.4 % [5].

Thus, with some justification, the rise in obesity prevalence, estimated by WHO to a number around half a billion adults, can be portrayed as a modern epidemic, given that statistical mapping over time illustrates something akin to a disease vector, now more apparent than ever as food and beverage corporations globalize their products and markets, exporting obesity – the "western disease" – to populations where it was scarcely known in the past. While obesity treatment is rarely successful in the long term, there are very few measures available to counteract the impact of obesity at a population level. At a strategic level, it has become clear that societies must learn to cope with the long-term consequences of having an obese population, placing significant additional demands on health services and with wider practical societal impacts. Thus, the challenge is now very much focused on finding how to prevent childhood obesity within an enduring socioeconomic structure that has demonstrably generated the levels of obesity we have today.

Given that rising obesity rates provide an indicator of population-wide weight gain, it is also apparent that the nature of the food chain has altered greatly for almost everyone. Although much of the alarm in the present-day food debate focuses on the manner in which agribusiness has forced the acceptance of genetically modified products with little concern for the uncertain health consequences, the change wrought over more than half century in the food chain through the predominance of processed foods, confectionery, and caloric drinks has created a dependence on virtually sterile foods with extended shelf lives, an excess of empty calories, and a deficit in fresh fruits and vegetables in the general diet, combined with an increasing detachment for many from an understanding of the origins of food and the healthiest nutritional combinations of those foods.

To some extent the debate is shifting from the obesity epidemic per se towards a self-defined group of noncommunicable diseases and related NGOs where there are close links with commercial interests. The International Diabetes Federation (IDF), for example, has courted controversy by accepting Nestlé as a sponsor, despite a long-standing campaign by some NGOs to boycott the company. Protests that the IDF is losing credibility have been voiced by distinguished figures in the field of diabetes research and public health [6].

The focus on noncommunicable diseases and their prevention, the basis of the 2011 UN General Assembly Resolution on the Prevention and Control of Noncommunicable Diseases (Resolution 66/2), has led to wider controversy about the closer involvement of major food and beverage sector corporations, along with some other sectors such as alcohol, with growing misgivings about conflicts of interest and the poor track record – and, in some cases, an outrageous history – of these companies wittingly or unwittingly frustrating progress in public health. A group of NGOs, led by the International Baby Food Action Network, have protested to the UN over NCD Alliance proposals for a "Global Coordinating Platform." They believe this would offer opportunities for industry stakeholders to take the lead as partners but argue that the UN's NCD resolution in 2011 did not provide for "collaboration with the private sector" [7].

Some see the NCD initiative as superseding the WHO's 2004 Global Strategy on Diet, Physical Activity and Health that witnessed the public health arena turned into a battleground in which there was no disguising the hostility of large parts of the food and beverage sector towards WHO's efforts to improve the food chain as one approach to tackling the obesity epidemic. Subsequently, many of the very small steps taken by a few governments have met with either overt or covert resistance.

In 2011 the US Federal Trade Commission's proposals for voluntary nutrition principles, tabled by its Interagency Working Group on Food Marketed to Children, were rejected by the food and beverage industries, leading the Institute of Medicine to reemphasize the need to address environmental cues rather than attribute blame to individuals and point to personal responsibility as the key to counteracting obesity [8]. Even the quite modest public health efforts of Mayor Michael

Bloomberg in New York City to moderate the excesses of the sugar drink consumption by simply limiting public venue serving sizes to 16 oz, or 1 pint, rather than the 32-oz or quart servings promoted by soda companies, encountered a very public hostile response from Coca-Cola and McDonald's before the very limited scope of this restriction came into force [9].

In practice, the impetus of worthwhile public health initiatives often ends up dissipated or diverted by commercial interests whose chief strategic concern has been to defeat any move towards effective regulation to control junk food and the marketing of such food, particularly to children. Companies simply switched the focus of their marketing to children from more expensive television advertising to exploit the much more targeted and substantially cheaper personalized marketing available via the Internet [10].

The frustratingly slow pace of achievement and implementation of any meaningful measures to prevent obesity proffers an unwelcome guarantee that the obesity epidemic is here to stay and will inevitably get worse. Whether or not it is now too late to address the challenge, only time will tell.

References

1. Eaton SB, Konner M, Shostak M. Stone agers in the fast lane: chronic degenerative diseases in evolutionary perspective. Am J Med. 1988;84(4):739–49.
2. Józsa L. Obesity in sculptures of the paleolithic era. Orv Hetil. 2008;149(49):2309–14.
3. Haslam D, Rigby N. A long look at obesity. Lancet. 2010; 376(9735):85–6.
4. OECD Health Data 2012 – frequently requested data. http://www.oecd.org/health/healthpoliciesanddata/oecdhealthdata2012-frequentlyrequesteddata.htm. Accessed 30 Sept 2012.
5. Gao Y, Ran X-W, Xie X-H, Lu H-L, Chen T, Ren Y, et al. Prevalence of overweight and obesity among Chinese Yi nationality: a cross-sectional study. BMC Public Health. 2011;11:919.
6. Beran D, Capewell S, de Courten M, Gale E, Gill G, Husseini A, et al. The International Diabetes Federation: losing its credibility by partnering with Nestlé? Lancet. 2012;380(9844):805.

7. Letter to the UN Secretary General: NGO Concerns about the proposal for a Global Coordination Platform on NCDs. http://info.babymilkaction.org/UNSG. 27 Sept 2012.

8. Glickman D, Parker L, Sim LJ, Del valle Cook H, Miller EA, editors. Accelerating progress in obesity prevention: solving the weight of the nation. Washington, DC: Committee on Accelerating Progress in Obesity Prevention, Food and Nutrition Board, Institute of Medicine of the National Academies; 2012.

9. Coke, McDonald's slam New York City bid to ban big soda cups REUTERS. New York. 2012. http://www.reuters.com/article/2012/05/31/us-usa-sugarban-reaction-idUS-BRE84U1BN20120531. Accessed 30 Sept 2012.

10. The 21st century gingerbread house. How companies are marketing junk food to children online. British Heart Foundation/Children's Food Campaign. http://www.bhf.org.uk/publications/view-publication.aspx?ps=1001772. 25 Dec 2011.

Chapter 3
Government Action to Tackle Obesity

Susan A. Jebb

Obesity is a "wicked" problem [1]. Excess weight gain is the end result of a network of determinants, each themselves the product of a wider set of individual, social, and environmental circumstances, exemplified by the obesity systems map developed by the UK Government Office for Science [2]. Obesity is everyone's problem, but it risks becoming no one's responsibility. Governments around the world have a vital leadership role to play in a number of key areas.

Making the Economic Case for Tackling Obesity

The systemic nature of the determinants of obesity is such that progress to reverse the problem will take time to yield positive health impacts. It is essential to have a clear understanding of the societal costs of inaction and the potential return on investment from interventions to prevent and treat obesity in order to justify investment, especially for costly capital projects such as environmental infrastructure.

S.A. Jebb, PhD
Human Nutrition Research,
Medical Research Council, 120 Fulbourn Road,
Cambridge, Cambridgeshire CB1 9NL, UK
e-mail: susan.jebb@mrc-hnr.cam.ac.uk

D.W. Haslam et al. (eds.), *Controversies in Obesity*,
DOI 10.1007/978-1-4471-2834-2_3,
© Springer-Verlag London 2014

Coordinating Action Across Government

While departments responsible for health will usually take the lead in efforts to treat obesity, many of the policy levers necessary for prevention lie in other government departments, including those responsible for business, education, transport, and welfare. It is vital that governments secure the cooperation of ministers to work across departmental boundaries to address all policies that directly or indirectly contribute to tackling obesity.

Working at an International Level to Secure Global Action

Some policies will be easier to implement, or be more effective, if enacted on a regional or global basis. This is particularly true for policies that require cooperation with globalized industries.

Monitoring Progress

Setting clear targets or other performance metrics provides a focus for action to reduce obesity. These may include changes in the key drivers of obesity, particularly diet and physical activity behaviors, as well as measurements of the prevalence of overweight and obesity. It is vital that governments put in place robust surveillance measures to provide regular feedback as part of a program of continuous learning to enhance public policies.

In recent years, most governments have recognized obesity as a public health problem, but their ability to take direct action to prevent or treat obesity among individual citizens is limited. Accordingly, governments need to work in partnership and to exert their influence through others using a mix of incentives and disincentives to motivate action. Increasingly this will be through local governance structures, building on evidence that local action, embedded in communities, is effective in preventing obesity [3]. Health care systems, too, need to be mobilized to recognize obesity as the root cause of a diverse range of health problems and encouraged to treat obesity as a key part of the management of chronic diseases [4]. Moreover, many people will be more likely to take action as a consequence of messaging from their peers, civil society groups, or trusted brands than from traditional authority figures.

In the UK, the Foresight report "Tackling Obesities: Future Choices" set out a framework for action across society, led by national government but working in partnership with others [2]. It provided an authoritative scientific review of the state of the evidence, with a strong policy focus. It has underpinned the development of two successive national strategies to tackle obesity in England, cutting across the political spectrum, and provided the backdrop to NICE guidance on tackling obesity at a local level [3]. It recommended an approach based on six key elements:

1. Systemic change across the system map, incorporating actions to address the full range of determinants of obesity
2. Complementary interventions at different levels: individual, local, national, and global
3. Interventions that touch individuals and populations at key points throughout the life course
4. A mixture of initiatives (focused policies which impose change), enablers (equipping individuals and communities with the skills to make changes), and amplifiers (population-level actions to shift social and cultural norms)
5. Short-, medium-, and long-term plans for change – recognizing that some policies may be essential prerequisites for other action, not least actions to build public acceptability for more paternalistic policies
6. Ongoing evaluation and continuous improvement to allow the strategy evolve as evidence of effectiveness accumulates

It is too early to judge the outcome of this strategy in England; while the rate of increase in obesity has slowed, or even halted in some age groups, a quarter of adults are obese and associated morbidity remains high [5]. It is apparent that in spite of substantial investment and effort in recent years, further action is still needed to accelerate progress. This includes continually reviewing and identifying gaps in the strategy, seeking more effective mechanisms to deliver changes, and securing global agreement on matters that are beyond the national jurisdiction.

But in a democracy, diet and activity habits are ultimately voluntary personal behaviors, and modern governments must respect the autonomy of their citizens. To this end, the Nuffield Council on Bioethics in Public Health proposed a stewardship model that "emphasises the obligation of states to provide conditions that allow people to be healthy and, in particular, to take measures to reduce health inequalities" [6]. It recognizes that interventions must be proportionate and proposes an intervention ladder to guide government action (Table 3.1). In order to tackle obesity, there is a broad agreement that action confined to the lower levels based around information and education is necessary but not sufficient, but there is currently little public acceptance of intrusive policies close to the top of the ladder that restrict choice except, on occasions, in the case of children where it is more readily accepted that the state has a stronger "duty of care." Thus, current policy discourse is focused towards the middle of the ladder, considering incentives and disincentives to change behavior, most notably policies involving changes in "choice architecture" [7] or fiscal measures [8].

Whether the balance of responsibility for tackling obesity rests with government, other actors, or individuals is a largely academic argument since progress will be maximized when all groups move in parallel. As more governments take on a strategic leadership role in tackling obesity, there will be opportunities to learn from a growing body of international experience, especially in the mechanisms to deliver effective policies. But a shift in social and cultural norms in the population towards

TABLE 3.1 The intervention ladder and its potential application to obesity policy

Eliminate choice: regulate in such a way as to entirely eliminate choice (e.g., banning confectionery in schools)

Restrict choice: regulate in such a way as to restrict the options available to people with the aim of protecting them (e.g., setting limits on fat or sugar content of food or drinks)

Guide choice through disincentives: fiscal and other disincentives can be put in place to influence people not to pursue certain activities (e.g., tax on sugar-sweetened drinks)

Guide choice through incentives: regulations can be offered that guide choices by fiscal and other incentives (e.g., schemes for the purchase of bicycles for journeys to work)

Guide choices through changing the default policy: regulations that make it easier to make the healthy choice (e.g., changing the default milk used in coffee shops to low-fat varieties)

Enable choice: policies that enable people to change to a healthier behavior (e.g., provision of clear nutritional labeling)

Provide information: inform and educate the public (e.g., campaigns to encourage people to take more exercise)

Do nothing or simply monitor the situation

Adapted from Nuffield Council on Bioethics [6]

valuing a healthy weight as a key element for future health will be a crucial element in developing a sustainable solution to obesity.

Conflicts of Interest SAJ was an independent Science Advisor on Obesity to the Department of Health in England (2007–2012) and is currently Chair of the Public Health Responsibility Deal Food Network.

References

1. Rutter H. Where next for obesity? Lancet. 2011;378(9793):746–7.
2. Butland B, Jebb SA, Kopelman P, McPherson K, Thomas S, Mardell J, et al. Foresight – tackling obesities: future choices – project report. London: Government Office for Science; 2007.

3. National Institute for Health and Clinical Excellence (NICE). Obesity: working with local communities, public health guidance 42. London: NICE; 2012.
4. Royal College of Physicians. Action on obesity: comprehensive care for all. Report of a working party. London: RCP; 2013.
5. Health Survey for England (HSE). Health and Social Care Information Centre. 2012. http://www.hscic.gov.uk/catalogue/PUB09300.
6. Nuffield Council on Bioethics. Public health: ethical issues. London: Nuffield Council on Bioethics; 2007.
7. Marteau TM, Ogilvie D, Roland M, Suhrcke M, Kelly MP. Judging nudging: can nudging improve population health? BMJ. 2011;342:d228.
8. Mytton OT, Clarke D, Rayner M. Taxing unhealthy food and drinks to improve health. BMJ. 2012;344:e2931.

Chapter 4
Why Are Governments Abdicating from Dealing with the Obesity Crisis?

Boyd A. Swinburn

Awareness and Actions on the Obesity Epidemic

The global patterns of obesity are fascinating. The beginnings of the epidemic can now be seen (retrospectively) to have started in the decades of the 1970s and 1980s in almost all the high- and middle-income countries [1], pointing to globalization factors, especially in food systems, as the overall drivers [2]. While the trajectories of the epidemics differ by country according to the existing food and physical activity environments upon which the global factors operated, there was a constant steep increase over the 1990s. This was a decade when researchers were trying to get the epidemic onto the public and political agendas. In the early 2000s, again virtually simultaneously across the globe, the media stories on obesity escalated exponentially [3]. So the question is: What have been the responses of the main players over the last decade to these increasing epidemics of both obesity and, more lately, media stories about obesity? A colleague who was responsible for the national nutrition survey in New Zealand in the 1990s, which showed this rapid rise in obesity,

B.A. Swinburn, MBChB, MD, FRACP
Section of Epidermiology and Biostatistics,
School of Population Health, University of Auckland,
261 Morrin St, Glen Innes, Auckland 1072, New Zealand
e-mail: boyd.swinburn@auckland.ac.nz

D.W. Haslam et al. (eds.), *Controversies in Obesity*,
DOI 10.1007/978-1-4471-2834-2_4,
© Springer-Verlag London 2014

explained the players thus: the researchers were the first runners in the "relay" and had done their job in showing the growing size of the problem and were ready to pass the baton to the policy makers. However, the policy makers were not yet in the stadium. The third relay runners, the politicians as the decision makers, did not even know that there was a race on. Meanwhile, the NGOs who were keen to run the last leg of the relay and do something about it were all stripped down and warmed up ready to go. The private sector groups, while not officially in the relay team, were rapidly gathering in the center of the stadium looking for opportunities to be involved in every leg of the race.

The two major players in influencing food environments are governments, because they have the authority to create the rules through policies and regulations, and the private sector, because they are already the major shapers of food environments and editors of consumer choices [4]. How have they responded to the obesity epidemic?

Responses of the Private Sector to the Obesity Epidemic

The transnational food companies have led a vigorous and rapid response to the perceived threat that the obesity epidemic poses to their businesses. While processed food as a product is different than tobacco as a product, the range of corporate responses from the large transnational food companies has followed and advanced the tactics used by the large tobacco companies in their fight against tobacco control measures. They have stepped up their lobbying of politicians to stall public health regulations [5] and to introduce industry-friendly regulations [6]; funded advertising campaigns and organizations against proposed public health regulations [7]; made general pledges to change their products and marketing practices [8]; instituted ineffective self-regulatory codes of practice [9]; funded industry-friendly scientists and research on physical activity [10]; funded non-regulatory approaches such as education and community action [11]; secured official roles within policy development committees and processes [12, 13]; formed "public private partnerships" with governments [14], NGOs [15], and professional bodies [16, 17]; and so on and on in what is rapidly becoming a truly comprehensive, tough-minded, multi-strategy, multi-sector approach.

Responses of the Public Sector to the Obesity Epidemic

Almost universally, governments have made a very slow response to the obesity epidemic. The potential reasons for this are manifold: the determinants are multiple and complex [18]; the potential solutions are multiple and contested, creating a "policy cacophony" [19]; there are no country-level exemplars of reversing obesity through public health action; there is scientific uncertainty about the optimal approaches; some solutions, such as social marketing and community interventions, cost significant ongoing funding; other solutions, such as restrictions on marketing, are heavily opposed by powerful, commercial interests; and still other solutions, such as endowing corporations with person status for the protection of free speech [20] or regulating when market forces fail, run counter to prevailing laws, cultures, and ideologies. Arguably the most important explanation for the extraordinary policy inaction of governments around the world is the very high level of political commitment and investment of "political capital" needed to institute policies that are so heavily opposed by powerful vested interests [21]. The leadership of Mayor Michael Bloomberg in securing policies to improve food and physical activity environments in New York City is a shining but rare example of strong government action [22]. In general, the level of collective political effort needed to pass "hard" policies (e.g., regulations to restrict unhealthy food marketing to children, taxes on unhealthy foods, or interpretive front-of-pack food labelling) is very high indeed, and there are many other political priorities and easier wins for politicians. However, doing nothing is increasingly untenable, and abdicating responsibilities to individuals, the marketplace, or "public private partnerships" is quickly proving to be just business as usual. What can be done to fortify the public policy-making process so that highly supported, evidence-informed, and effective policies can be implemented?

Lifting Government Actions to Prevent Obesity

There are actions that can help to protect public policy making from undue commercial-interest pressure and to increase the public demand for action, including:

- *Reducing conflicts of interest the policy-making process.* There should be no place at the table for individuals with high conflicts of interest between commercial and public good outcomes. For example, peak lobby groups for processed food companies should be considered too conflicted to sit on committees developing dietary guidelines, health claims regulations, food labelling requirements, and so on. They have a very legitimate role, however, in being involved in policy implementation.
- *Increasing the transparency in policy making and commercial lobbying efforts.* Lobby registers, required declarations of meetings between politicians and lobbyists, full declaration of party political donations, strong freedom of information laws, ready public access, and input into policy making are all important systems to help ensure that commercial influences on public policies are transparent and minimized.
- *Evidence and benchmarking.* Research and monitoring that show the level of progress in obesity prevention actions compared to international benchmarks will help to set standards and targets for policy making, especially towards creating healthier food environments.

- *Public pressure for action.* Public advocacy efforts to promote public policies could be strengthened by linking with allied movements such as those for environmental sustainability, food sovereignty, animal welfare, urban liveability, and social justice [23].

Conclusion

Current government responses to the obesity epidemic fall very far short of being commensurate with the size and seriousness of the problem. This inaction over decades is likely to be due, in large part, to the excessive influences of the commercial sector on public policy development. Major changes in policy processes and power dynamics will be needed to achieve government action that will shift us away from the current business as usual course and its consequent rises in obesity.

References

1. World Health Organization. Global status report on noncommunicable diseases 2010. Geneva: World Health Organization; 2011.
2. Swinburn BA, Sacks G, Hall KD, McPherson K, Finegood DT, Moodie ML, et al. The global obesity pandemic: shaped by global drivers and local environments. Lancet. 2011;378(9793): 804–14.
3. Rowe S. Global trends in obesity-related media coverage. Nutr Today. 2004;39(6):256.
4. Cohen DA, Babey SH. Contextual influences on eating behaviours: heuristic processing and dietary choices. Obes Rev. 2012;13(9): 766–79.
5. Corporate Europe Observatory. A red light for consumer information: the food industry's €1-billion campaign to block health warnings on food: Corporate Europe Observatory. 2010. Available from: http://corporateeurope.org/sites/default/files/sites/default/files/files/article/CEO-Food-Labelling.pdf. Cited 31 Oct 2012.
6. Personal Responsibility in Food Consumption Act of 2005, H.R. 554, 109th Congress. 2005.
7. Center for Responsive Politics. Lobbyists representing American Beverage Assn: Center for Responsive Politics. Available from:

http://www.opensecrets.org/lobby/clientlbs.php?id=D000000491&y ear=2010. Cited 31 Oct 2012.

8. Healthy Weight Commitment Foundation. Healthy Weight Commitment Foundation Overview: Healthy Weight Commitment Foundation. Available from: http://www.healthyweightcommit.org/ about/overview/. Cited 31 Oct 2012.

9. Australian Communications and Media Authority. Industry self-regulation of food and beverage advertising to children: ACMA monitoring report. Canberra: Australian Communications and Media Authority. 2011. Available from: http://www.acma.gov.au/ webwr/_assets/main/lib310132/industry_self-regulation-advertising_ to_children_monitoring_report-dec2011.pdf.

10. The Coca-Cola Company. Physical activity for health: what kind? How much? How intense?: the Coca Cola Company. Updated Jan 2012. Available from: http://www.beverageinstitute.org/en_us/pages/ expert-physical-activity-steven-blair.html. Cited 31 Oct 2012.

11. Nestlé. Supporting obesity-prevention programmes, EPODE: Nestlé. 2012. Available from: http://www.nestle.com/csv/ CreatingSharedValueCaseStudies/AllCaseStudies/Pages/ Supporting-obesity-prevention-programmes.aspx. Cited 31 Oct 2012.

12. Nestle M. Food politics: how the food industry influences nutrition and health. Berkeley: University of California Press; 2002.

13. Physicians Committee for Responsible Medicine. Court Rules Against USDA's secrecy and failure to disclose conflict of interest in setting nutrition policies. Washington, DC: Physicians Committee for Responsible Medicine; 2000. Available from: http://www.pcrm.org/ search/?cid=1162. Cited 31 Oct 2012.

14. UK Department of Health. Public health responsibility deal: our partners: UK Department of Health. Available from: http://responsi-bilitydeal.dh.gov.uk/our-partners/. Cited 31 Oct 2012.

15. Save the Children Federation. Corporate partners. Westport CT: Save the Children; 2012. Available from: http://www.savethechildren. org/site/c.8rKLIXMGIpI4E/b.6148397/k.C77B/Corporate_Partners. htm. Cited 31 Oct 2012.

16. Nestlé. Nestlé contributes to fight against non-communicable diseases: Nestlé; 2012. Available from: http://www.nestle.com/Media/ NewsAndFeatures/Pages/Diabetes-partnership.aspx. Cited 31 Oct 2012.

17. Deardorff J. Critics pounce on Coke, Pepsi health initiatives: skeptics chide health groups for taking money from makers of sugary drinks, fatty foods. Chicago: Tribune; 2012. Available from: http:// articles.chicagotribune.com/2012-02-05/news/ct-met-coke-pepsi-health-20120205_1_coca-cola-north-america-health-groups-healthy-lifestyle-choices. Cited 31 Oct 2012.

18. Butland B, Jebb S, Kopelman P, McPherson K, Thomas S, Mardell J, et al. Foresight: tackling obesities: future choices – project report. Department of Innovation Universities and Skills; 2007. Available from: http://www.bis.gov.uk/assets/foresight/docs/obesity/17.pdf.
19. Lang T, Rayner G. Overcoming policy cacophony on obesity: an ecological public health framework for policymakers. Obes Rev. 2007;8 Suppl 1:165–81.
20. Tucker A. Flawed assumptions: a corporate law analysis of free speech and corporate personhood in *Citizens United*. No. 2011-06. Georgia State University College of Law Legal Studies Research Paper; 2011.
21. Hastings G. Why corporate power is a public health priority. Br Med J. 2012;345:e5124.
22. Kliff S. Mayor Mike Bloomberg, public health autocrat: a brief history. Washington Post. 2012. Available from: http://www.washingtonpost.com/blogs/ezra-klein/post/mayor-mike-bloomberg-public-health-autocrat-a-brief-history/2012/06/04/gJQArSJbDV_blog.html. Cited 31 Oct 2012.
23. Robinson TN. Save the world, prevent obesity: piggybacking on existing social and ideological movements. Obesity. 2010;18 Suppl 1:S17–22.

Chapter 5
Childhood Habits and the Obesity Epidemic

Michael E.J. Lean

However it is assessed, the prevalence of obesity has clearly risen recently in all countries, and in general it is continuing to rise, even in the countries with the highest current obesity prevalences. This has brought colossal, new, and, in principle, avoidable health-care and social costs. Almost all those costs arise from obesity in adulthood, and from secondary consequences of obesity, rather than treatment costs.

In the hunt for causes, or perhaps scapegoats, it has become usual to focus attention on the rise in overweight or "obesity" in childhood. Many assume that the very evident increase in numbers of overweight children, visibly different from previous generations in the playground, is a direct causative forerunner to the rise in adult obesity. However, the rise in prevalence of obesity in childhood did not predate the rise in adults and it is more likely that the increase in overweight and obese children is a result of diet and activity changes in parents, in an industry-led epidemic which affects all age groups.

M.E.J. Lean, MA, MD, BChir
School of Medicine, MVLS, Human Nutrition,
University of Glasgow, Walton Building, Royal Infirmary,
84 Castle Street, Glasgow G4 0SF, UK
e-mail: mike.lean@glasgow.ac.uk

D.W. Haslam et al. (eds.), *Controversies in Obesity*,
DOI 10.1007/978-1-4471-2834-2_5,
© Springer-Verlag London 2014

Obesity is a pervasive disease, with multiple costly clinical consequences, which accumulate with age. As well as the closely related major metabolic and physical consequences, obese adults have increased number of "minor" ailments and take more time off work (Table 5.1). They visit general practitioners more often, with a range of symptoms (much more commonly over the age of about 40) and go on to develop disabling physical and metabolic diseases secondary to their obesity. Extreme obesity (e.g., BMI >50) is much more frequent in women and among the most deprived populations sectors. Severe obesity is the most rapidly growing category, and the most expensive, with substantially more medical and social costs than more modest obesity (e.g., BMI 30–40). The conventional BMI cutoff of 30 for "obesity" was

TABLE 5.1 Medical consequences of overweight and obesity are all multifactorial and age-related, and few develop in childhood

Physical symptoms	Metabolic	Social
Tiredness	Hypertension	Isolation
Breathlessness	NIDDM	Agoraphobia
Varicose veins	Hepatic steatosis	Unemployment
Back pain	Hyperlipidemia	Family/marital stress
Arthritis	Hypercoagulation	Discrimination
Edema/cellulitis	IHD and stroke	Financial
Sweating/intertrigo		
Stress incontinence		

Anesthetic/surgical	Endocrine	Psychological
Sleep apnea	Hirsutism	Low self-esteem
Chest infections	Oligomenorrhea/infertility	Self-deception
Wound dehiscence	Metromenorrhea	Cognitive disturbance
Hernia	Estrogen dependent	Distorted body image
Venous thrombosis	Cancers: breast, uterus, prostate, colorectal	Depression

established for epidemiological purposes and is often mis-leading in clinical settings and when applied to individuals. Fit rugby players and other athletes commonly have BMI 30–35, with low body fat content. Waist circumference >102 cm in men, or >88 cm in women, is a better guide to excess body fat, and to increased medical costs, which demand professional intervention. These figures only apply to adults. Waist cut-offs are not so well defined for fat children.

As the obesity epidemic has unfolded in adults, with colos-sal cost burdens for health care and insurance premiums, there has been a parallel increase in the prevalence of over-weight children. UK and US anti-obesity strategies have placed enormous emphasis on the rise in "childhood obesity." Is this truly the cause of adult obesity, or a consequence of it? How much does the increase in so-called childhood obesity actually matter?

A crude analysis of government reports and strategy ini-tiatives against obesity reveals that around half of the total national effort against obesity has been directed against chil-dren, much of it specifically for interventions in schools. Why has this emphasis arisen? Is that the priority for our very limited resources?

In the UK, for example, the most recent White Paper on Public Health for England [1] sets a target for reducing "childhood obesity" (at age 11), but none for adults. The 2008 UK Cross-Government Obesity Strategy reiterates the pri-mary target to reduce childhood obesity and includes nine action points directed at children, eight general actions, and only two directed specifically at adults with obesity [2]. The NICE guideline includes four pages on preventing childhood obesity, compared with two specifically on adults [3]. The US Surgeon General's Office launched a prominent specific ini-tiative for childhood overweight and obesity prevention in 2007 [4]. The underpinning thinking behind this focus is a belief-based view that preventing childhood obesity will lead to lifelong behavioral changes, and ultimately to arresting the epidemic of (adult) obesity. Evidence-based detractors have pointed out that over 80 % of obese adults were not overweight as children [5–7] and that the tracking of overweight/obesity and of physical activity pattern, from childhood into adulthood, is weak until teenage years [8]. Furthermore, "obese" children, as commonly defined (BMI >95th or even >98th centile for 1990), are mostly only "overweight," not "obese," when they reach the age of 16–18 years (Fig. 5.1) [9]. Using the more appropriate international data, linked to BMI in adulthood, far fewer children are classified as "obese" (Fig. 5.2) [9]. There is no evidence that preventing childhood obesity will reduce subsequent adult obesity, which is where virtually all health consequences and costs lie, and the evidence for efficacy, effectiveness, or cost-effectiveness of interventions for childhood obesity is weak, lacking, or negative [10, 11]. We can learn from these studies directed at children, and build on successful elements, but the focus looks fundamentally flawed.

A functionalist definition of "epidemic" is a prevalence of disease which has risen above the level which can be contained using conventional 1:1 medical services, and above which political, preventive action is demanded. An epidemic

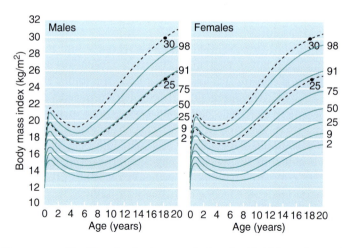

FIGURE 5.1 Gentiles for body mass index for British males and females. Gentile curves are spaced two thirds of z score apart. Also shown are body mass index values of 25 and 30 kg/m² at age 18, with extra centile curves drawn through them

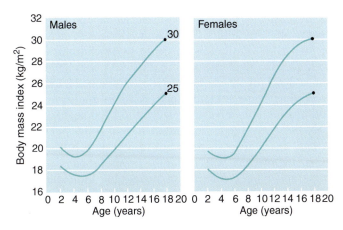

FIGURE 5.2   International cut off points for body mass index by sex for overweight and obesity, passing through body mass index 25 and 30 kg/m² at age 18 (data from Brazil, Britain, Hong Kong, Netherlands, Singapore, and United States)

is thus both a medical and a political responsibility, combining optimal patient care (within resource limits) with effective population-directed preventive measures.

Obesity shares common features with many diseases that doctors have to treat, but it has several very specific characteristics that demand different approaches. Obesity has become "normal" for many people, and researchers have produced evidence that obese children are mostly not recognized as having a serious disease by their parents [12, 13]. Perhaps that is actually acceptable. Campaigns to raise awareness of "childhood obesity," for example, through schools health service examinations [14, 15] have met with antagonism. Children classified as "obese" according to current criteria are mostly not ill, in any other definable sense, and do not occupy GP surgeries more than thinner children. Indeed one American study found that obese children actually had lower health-care costs than thinner ones [16]. The tracking of obesity from childhood is weak. Children classified as overweight or obese, under the age of 10, have little increased risk of adult obesity [8], but obese teenagers are likely to become obese as adults. However, when "obese children" on the 98th BMI-centile-for-age cease to be children (at 16 in Scotland, 18 in England, or 21 in the USA), they actually only have a BMI of 27–28 kg/m². They are mostly overweight (exceptions being athletes such as rugby players) but still need to gain quite a bit more weight to become "obese."

Excess body fat in childhood is not good, but isolated extreme cases apart, it does not impair physical health. As adults, overweight will certainly promote metabolic syndrome and type 2 diabetes in susceptible individuals, even before those individuals become "obese" (qua BMI >30), and a range of other metabolic and physical problems. But "obese" children will not suffer the full consequences of obesity without extra adult weight gain. The normal insulin resistance of puberty can result in impairment of glucose tolerance which reaches the diagnostic threshold for type 2 diabetes in some very obese teenagers, but the numbers are small, and this is a transient biochemical phenomenon usually with no health impairment.

There is evidence that overweight/obese children have increased number of minor psychological difficulties than normal-weight children, and they have been shown to have poorer educational and career prospects and are less likely to have stable domestic status [17]. So there are good reasons to want to help overweight/obese children to control their weights. It is important, however, to recognize that this is not the only, or most important, solution to national obesity epidemic.

That being the case, we need to know what is causing more children to become obese now. Several factors are fairly consistent and make sense. It has been known for many years that obese children are likely to have overweight/obese parents. That could point to genetic factors, but the association is very strong, whereas genetic factors behind obesity are insufficient to explain it. The most authoritative evidence base, the gene map of obesity [18], suggests that about 20–30 % of variance in BMI is explained by genetic factors. The greater part is environmental. Interestingly, studies of "heritability" of BMI among twins, comparing BMI status of identical and non-identical twins, always suggest a much higher heritable influence than other types of studies. This is not fully explained: the very close similarity of identical twins is partly genetic but also may reflect the parental habit of treating identical twins identically, so adding identical environmental pressures. On the other hand, parents may tend to treat their non-identical twins differently as a matter of principle, so generating greater differences than would usually be expected between like-sex siblings at the same age.

There is growing interest in the possibility of epigenetic effects, such that an obese woman who overeats in pregnancy may induce lifelong epigenetic changes in the appetite control of a fetus. In animal models this appears more marked for female offspring, possibly exploring the greater likelihood of obesity in the daughters of obese mothers [19]. The alternative explanation is of old-fashioned behavioral direction between mothers and daughters, fathers and sons [20].

Government strategies against any epidemic must attempt to achieve a total funding level appropriate to the clinical care burdens, modified by voters' likely assessment of the actions taken. The strategy needs to apportion funding between effective and sustainable measures for prevention and for treatment of affected individuals within available budgets. The evidence on treating obesity is rather different in children from that in adults.

As far as prevention goes, it is probably fair to say that we do not have any model for intervention which has proven effectiveness, either for adults or children. A recent evaluation of attempts to prevent excessive weight gain in children concluded that there was no cost-effective method within current evidence. Interventions aimed at increasing physical activity have been popular (e.g., in schools). The results show almost total failure to modify children's BMI centiles, probably because children who exercise more in school compensate by inactivity out of school [21]. While some interventions suggest small reductions in body fat during the intervention itself, any such effect is lost within 1 month after the end of the exercise program, and there is no evidence that preventing "childhood obesity" will reduce later adult obesity [22].

No country has yet produced a convincing down-turn in rising adult national obesity prevalences. There are recent suggestions from UK that could indicate such a decline [23]. Even if the heights and weights data do show a flattening or down-turn in numbers with BMI >30, there remains a steep rise in numbers with BMI >40 and >50, which is where the big problems are. It also seems that waist circumferences are continuing to rise steeply, even when BMI is rising less, probably indicating rapid accumulation of body fat while muscle mass has declined [23]. To make it difficult to monitor what is happening in the population, the dietary methods and waist circumference method used in the Health Survey of England and Scottish Health Surveys have recently been changed, so the data are confounded by differences in survey methods and different sampling methods. It thus becomes impossible to obtain reliable longitudinal data, either for waist circumference or for the dietary factors which might be influential in any change [23]. It is deplorable that the commissioners of national surveys have failed to understand the very basic principle that longitudinal surveys need to use consistent protocols and methods.

In relation to obesity treatment, the evidence is more secure. We now have growing evidence for efficacy and cost-effectiveness for obesity treatment programs available in the NHS, with results at 12 months as called for by NICE and SIGN guidelines. It has long been clear, and accepted, that no obesity treatment can be effective for all patients and that a substantial proportion of obese patients will always fail to engage or lose weight. A recent systematic review of UK data has established that about 30 % of patients will engage, with variable levels of success such that about half of those (i.e., 15 % of all starters) can maintain a weight loss >5 %. This generalization applies to first-level "self-help" approached using commercial slimming clubs and to the next level of 1:1 professional input provided in routine primary care by

Counterweight [24]. The evidence is not yet secure for the multidisciplinary secondary-care methods used for the next stage (e.g. by Glasgow and Clyde Weight Management Service), although 3-month results are encouraging. For severe and complicated obesity, a low-energy liquid diet approach delivered by practice nurses in routine primary care can generate and maintain for 12 months >15 kg weight loss for about 33 % of patients [25]. None of these results are perfect, and there is scope for future improvement, but it is valuable that these data have been obtained from largely unselected patients in real-life settings, rather than in the artificial context of randomized controlled trials.

Among obese children, results have been much less positive. Systematic reviews have found only weak evidence for interventions to treat childhood obesity [26]. Physical activity interventions are particularly poorly sustained in childhood [22]. The much-quoted high-input interventions of Epstein, unfeasible for routine use, were effective with the involvement of parents. A number of more recent studies have also documented the importance of involving parents, and several have now suggested that interventions that involve solely parents are effective against the obesity of children. There are several aspects to this, including attention to parenting skills and styles, but is seems possible that children with weight problems are following the ill-advised diets and lifestyles of their overweight parents. If parents set a better example, including controlling their own weight problems, then it is possible that children will follow suit and potentially adopt diets and lifestyles compatible with a lifelong normal body weight.

Children's eating and physical activity habits are likely to be influenced more by parents, or other household members, than by any others. Schools certainly have potential to educate, and a useful basic understanding of energy balance and the energy and nutrient contents of food groups can be taught in primary schools. School meals provide an opportunity to demonstrate attractive meals which satisfy the basic principles of nutrition defined by the Caroline

Walker Trust [27], and now adopted nationally with (or despite?) the antics of certain celebrity chefs. All too often, however, the quest for short-term profitability on very low budgets, coupled with inadequate training in nutrition among caterers, has led to poor-quality school meals and continued failure to provide a nutritionally balanced meal for schoolchildren. Extraordinarily, the UK government has suggested not applying nutritional standards for the new free school and academies, following a similar move by the New Zealand Government. Who benefits from that? Children deserve better. Under UNICEF declaration, every child has a right to clean air, clean water, and nutritious food [28].

Even with proper training and commitment, and perhaps a larger budget, school meals themselves will not solve childhood obesity: maximally 5 a week for 40 weeks – 200 meals a year is a relatively small proportion of the 1,200 or so eating occasions each child will negotiate. Similarly, the evidence is increasingly clear that physical activity in schools cannot be sufficient to habitualize physical activity such that it will persist past the age 11 watershed into secondary school age and adulthood. The role of parents in normalizing either regular physical activity or inactivity is likely to be much greater. The problem is likely to be one of degree. Most young adults rate themselves as reasonably active ("never off my feet"), but when actually measured, their physical activity level is revealed to be very low. It is worth reflecting that humans, as a species, scarcely experienced obesity throughout millions of years of evolution until in recent decades it became possible to live without working physically. Evidence using step-counters has indicated that in order to avoid all cardiovascular risk factors and overweight, humans may need to walk for about 4 h daily, amassing over 15,000 steps per day, and spend about 7 h a day in upright posture [29]. That is probably the level of activity undertaken by most people through evolution, and for which our bodies and appetites evolved. By secondary school age, that is the sort of level that should be normal for human beings, not just a nebulous target.

References

1. Choosing health: making healthy choices easier. 2004. http://www.dh.gov.uk/en/Publicationsandstatistics/Publications/PublicationsPolicyandGuidance/DH_4094550. Accessed Feb 2013.
2. Healthy Weight, Healthy Lives. A cross government strategy for England. 2008. http://www.dh.gov.uk/en/Publicationsandstatistics/Publications/PublicationsPolicyandGuidance/DH_082378. Accessed Feb 2013.
3. NICE. Obesity: the prevention, identification, assessment and management of overweight and obesity in adults and children. 2006. http://www.nice.org.uk/CG43. Accessed Feb 2013.
4. US Office of the Surgeon General. Overweight in children and adolescents. 2007. http://www.surgeongeneral.gov/topics/obesity/calltoaction/fact_adolescents.htm. Accessed Feb 2013.
5. Herman KM, Craig CL, Gauvin L, Katzmarzyk PT. Tracking of obesity and physical activity from childhood to adulthood: the physical activity longitudinal study. Int J Pediatric Obes. 2008;15:1–8.
6. Deshmukh-Taskar P, Nicklas TA, Morales M, Yang SJ, Zakeri I, Berenson GS. Tracking of overweight status from childhood to young adulthood: the Bogalusa Heart Study. Eur J Clin Nutr. 2006;60:48–57.
7. Janssen I, Katzmaryzyk PT, Srinivasan SR, Chen W, Malina RM, Bouchard C, et al. Utility of childhood BMI in the prediction of adulthood disease: comparison of national and international references. Obes Res. 2005;13:1106–15.
8. Singh AS, Mulder C, Twisk JW, van Mechelen W, Chinapaw MJ. Tracking of childhood overweight into adulthood: a systematic review of the literature. Obes Res. 2008;9:474–88.
9. Cole T, Bellizzi MC, Flegal KM. Establishing a standard definition for child overweight and obesity worldwide: international survey. BMJ. 2000;320:1–6.
10. Taylor RW, McAuley KA, Barbezat W, Farmer VL, Williams SM, Mann JI. Two-year follow-up of an obesity prevention initiative in children: the APPLE project. Am J Clin Nutr. 2008;88:1371–7.
11. Hughes AR, Stewart L, Chapple J, McColl JH, Donaldson MD, Kelnar CJ, et al. Randomized, controlled trial of a best-practice individualized behavioral program for treatment of childhood overweight: Scottish Childhood Overweight Treatment Trial (SCOTT). Pediatrics. 2008;121:e539–46.
12. White A, O'Brien B, Houlihan T, Darker C, O'Shea B. Childhood obesity: parents fail to recognise, general practitioners fail to act. Ir Med J. 2012;105(1):10–3.
13. Worcester S. Parents may fail to recognise overweight, obesity as problem in kids. http://www.pediatricnews.com/cme/click-for-credit-articles/single-article/parents-may-fail-to-recognize-overweight-

obesity-as-problem-in-kids/665f619f07bae6e53b91d68b98f26bfb. html. Accessed Feb 2013.

14. Puhl RM, Heuer CA. Obesity stigma: important considerations for public health. Am J Public Health. 2010;100(6):1019–28.

15. Childhood obesity campaign still bullying fat kids. http://bitchmagazine.org/post/childhood-obesity-campaign-still-bullying-fat-kids. Accessed Feb 2013

16. John J, Wenig CM, Wolfenstetter SB. Recent economic findings on childhood obesity: cost-of-illness and cost-effectiveness of interventions. Curr Opin Clin Nutr Metab Care. 2010;13(3):305–13.

17. Sweeting H, Anderson A, West P. Socio-demographic correlates of dietary habits in mid to late adolescence. Eur J Clin Nutr. 1994;48(10): 736–48.

18. Bouchard C, Perusse L. Current status of the human obesity gene map. Obes Res. 1996;4(1):81–90.

19. Perez-Pastor EM, Metcalf BS, Hosking J, Jeffery AN, Voss LD, Wilkin TJ. Assortative weight gain in mother-daughter and father-son pairs: an emerging source of childhood obesity. Longitudinal study of trios (EarlyBird 43). Int J Obes (Lond). 2009;33:727–35.

20. Lean MEJ. Childhood obesity: time to shrink a parent. Int J Obes (Lond). 2010;34:1–3.

21. Fremeaux AE, Mallam KM, Metcalf BS, Hosking J, Voss LD, Wilkin TJ. The impact of school-time activity on total physical activity: the activitystat hypothesis (Early Bird 46). Int J Obes (Lond). 2011; 35(10):1277–83.

22. Metcalf BS, Henley W, Wilkin T. Effectiveness of intervention on physical activity of children: a systematic review and meta-analysis of controlled trials with objectively measured outcomes (EarlyBird 54). BMJ. 2012;27:345.

23. Lean MEJ, Katsarou C, McLoone P, Morrison D. Changes in BMI and waist circumference in Scottish adults: use of repeated cross-sectional surveys to explore multiple age groups and birth-cohorts. Int J Obes (Lond). 2013;37(6):800–8.

24. McCombie L, Lean MEJ, Haslam D and the Counterweight team. Effective UK weight management services for adults. Clin Obes. 2012;2:96–102.

25. Lean MEJ, Brosnahan N, McLoone P, McCombie L, Bell-Higgs A, Ross H, et al. Feasibility and indicative results from a 12-month Low-Energy-Liquid-Diet treatment and maintenance programme for severe obesity. Br J Gen Pract. 2013;63(607):115–24.

26. Summerbell CD, Ashton V, Campbell KJ, Edmunds L, Kelly S, Waters E. Interventions for treating obesity in children. Cochrane Database Syst Rev. 2003;3:CD001872.

27. Eating well at school. Nutritional and practical guidelines. The Caroline Walker Trust. 2005. http://www.cwt.org.uk/pdfs/ EatingWellatSchool.pdf. Accessed Feb 2013

28. UNICEF rights for every child. http://www.unicef.org/rightsite/files/rightsforeverychild.pdf. Accessed Feb 2013.
29. Tigbe W. Patterns of free-living physical activity and posture. Objective measurement and relation to coronary risk. PhD thesis. Caledonian University, Glasgow. 2009.

Chapter 6
Obesity and Sexuality

David W. Haslam

Some commentators have suggested that obesity and intercourse are poorly compatible. In 1972, *The Joy of Sex* stated: "If you are grossly overweight, set about losing it, whether you value your sex life or only your life," suggesting entry from the rear and intercourse on hard surfaces as solutions. A study of obesity and sexual quality of life [1], among 507 obese people seeking treatment and 422 obese and 282 normal-weight participants not actively seeking help, concluded that obesity impairs sexual activity compared with healthy weight. The fat acceptance organization Dimensions disagrees, publishing a guide to enhanced sexual relationships and positions, beginning "The Mythology of Obesity tells us that sex with a fat partner is either fruitless or impossible" but continues: "In the real world, sex is more likely to be impeded by anxiety than adiposity." Suggested positions in addition to traditional acts include the upside-down position, the T-square and X positions, and stand and deliver. The latter was apparently beloved of Edward VII, who commissioned a chair in 1890, his "siege d'amour" to facilitate the act [2] with prostitutes at the opulent brothel Le Chabanais, one of the great bordellos of *fin de siècle* Paris (Fig. 6.1). The chair allowed him to "leverage himself"

D.W. Haslam, MBBS, DGM
Doctor's Surgery, Watton Place Clinic,
60 High Street, Watton at Stone, SG143SY, UK
e-mail: dwhaslam@aol.com

D.W. Haslam et al. (eds.), *Controversies in Obesity*,
DOI 10.1007/978-1-4471-2834-2_6,
© Springer-Verlag London 2014

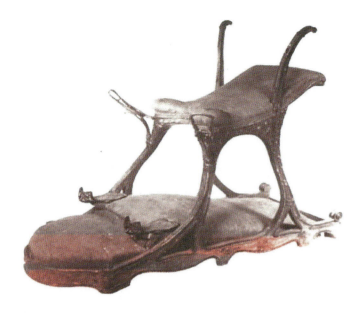

FIG. 6.1 Edward VII's "siege d'amour"

from the wheelbarrow style arms "while thrusting." His partner or partners were thus protected from being crushed by the Prince's excess weight [3].

Dimensions Forum reveals sexual practices unique to obese individuals. One contributor advised: "I adore BBW's and SSBBW's [big beautiful woman, and super-sized big beautiful woman] as well and LOVE their soft bellies and the rolls that go along with them … a belly jiggling as a girl is having sex." Many describe the "belly f**k" and other erotic and autoerotic practices. "I LOVE when my belly hangs over my pants, and I can rub it and feel how big it is. I love to get my fingers all the way under the hang and pick it up and jiggle so I can feel how heavy the bottom roll is."

There are important ethnic considerations, sometimes concerning peripheral adiposity and body morphology. According to Professor Myra Mendible, "In mainstream U.S. culture, 'bubble butts' have typically been associated with 'lowly' subject positions or 'vulgar' sexuality. Calling too much attention to one's behind is considered uncouth in polite society, a nasty reminder of forbidden or distasteful acts. A big butt is associated with 'unnatural' sex, excrement, or the excess and physicality identified with 'darker' races."

However, within the Black community larger female body types have long been admired: "No one wants a bone but a dog!" Recently, more and more Americans are lauding the "gluteal aesthetic" thanks to "bootylicious" celebrities such as J. Lo and Beyoncé, and the "butt" has become a means of celebrating rather than condemning ethnic differences, and for some, signalling an invitation to sexual pleasure. Gluteal implants exist to enhance the less well-endowed rear. Rapper Sir Mix-A-Lot recorded "Baby Got Back," revealing his fondness for a "big butt" and its ethnic association:

> I mean, her butt, is just so big.
> I can't believe it's just so round, it's like,
> out there, I mean—gross. Look!
> She's just so … black!
> I like big butts and I can not lie
> You other brothers can't deny
> That when a girl walks in with an itty bitty waist
> And a round thing in your face

Even Frank Zappa in "Sex" sang: "The bigger the cushion, the better the pushin." The expression "phat" has been coined by hip-hop African-American culture, meaning, variously "pretty, hot, and tempting" or "pussy, hips, and tits," to glorify bigger women. Many rappers themselves have been obese, often morbidly so, such as Biggie Smalls, aka Notorious B. I. G., who weighed 395 lb when he was shot dead in Los Angeles in 1997. Size was often displayed as hyper-maleness.

Thin Men and Big Women

Psychologist Mildred Klingman explains the sexual dynamics whereby an ordinary man might prefer a fat woman. "There are many such men…. 'Sure I like 'em big. I don't want to have to shake the sheets to find my woman.'" The display of

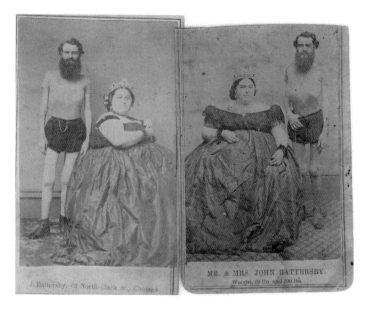

MR. & MRS. JOHN BATTERSBY.
Weight, 69 lbs. and 700 lbs.

J. Battersby, 63 North Clark St., Chicago.

Fig. 6.2 Mr. and Mrs. John Battersby

fat for sexual pleasure first reached a peak in Victorian times; circus fat ladies of the era were "the most erotically appealing of all freaks, with the possible exception of male dwarfs." One of the first circus fat ladies of the modern era was Hannah Crouse, who began her career in 1859, eventually weighing around 800 lb and married the famous "human skeleton" John Battersby (Fig. 6.2).

In contrast....

Feeders and Feedees

A person who gains arousal by being fed is a "feedee," the person providing the substrate a "feeder," although the feeder-feedee relationship may not always be overtly sexual, but nonetheless has sexual undercurrents. The ultimate expression of commitment between a feeder and a feedee is for the latter to achieve "immobility," thereby relying exclusively on the former, as a baby to its mother both in utero and in infancy. Supersize Betsy is a feedee who weighed over 500 lb when interviewed by the journal RE/search but claimed to be waiting for the right man before attempting to achieve immobility. "I wouldn't want to put it on casually." She claims, with regard to her many admirers, that "All of them—down to the very last one—have some kind of fantasy of me sitting on top of them or laying on top of them or just enveloping them. To them, it's like being smothered in chocolate syrup. It's not a death wish or suffocation thing—it's more about being able to feel this femininity surrounding you completely.... Us feedees are sexually pretty selfish, because we just want to lay there and be pampered and fed and adored and worshipped." Jeb, who is a feeder, or "encourager," finds female fat comforting—"like a big, soft feather bed I can fall asleep on." He says he likes to nuzzle his face in his girlfriend's teats and belly. He speaks hopefully of a day when he'll be able to get "swallowed up in her fat" as if she were an amoeba and he was a food particle [4]. The American group the National Association for the Advancement of Fat Acceptance (NAAFA) [5] exists "to help build a society in which people of every size are accepted with dignity and equality in all aspects of life." It has an official policy against feederism, stating that "NAAFA supports an individual's right to control all choices concerning his or her own body. NAAFA opposes the practice of feeders, in which one partner in a sexual relationship expects and encourages another partner to gain weight.... That all bodies, of all sizes, are joyous and that individuals of all sizes can and should expect and demand respect from sexual partners for their bodies just as they are. That people of all sizes become empowered to demand respect for their bodies in the context of sexual relationships, without attempting to lose or gain weight in order to win a partner's approval or attract or retain that partner's desire" [6].

Gay Aspects and Perceptions

Cookie Woolner, a burlesque performer with the Original Fat-Bottom Review and the Chainsaw Chubbettes, agrees that fat is erotic: "By taking off a corset to reveal my tummy while dancing confidently and seductively as it shakes, my actions express more than words ... and gives everyone in the audience permission to expand their definitions of beauty beyond what we've been taught. Queer fat burlesque shows us new possibilities for how to live in our bodies." FaT GiRL, a San Francisco lesbian journal which celebrated "Fat Dykes and the Women who Want Them," bracketed alongside other "alternative" sexual scenarios, showing big women with tattoos and piercings engaged in sadomasochistic situations, while erotically feeding each other, promoting fat bodies over and above the body morphology of their smaller sisters.

For men, it is very different. An obese man is sometimes considered to have lost his masculinity; instead of being chiselled and hard, he is soft and rounded, with androgynous "moobs" or "man breasts" where chest hair has disappeared due to friction with his clothes. In the journal "Rump Parliament," in contrast, Daniel Pinkwater explains how his "globularity" implied lack of unpleasant typically male "A-type, killer-instinct, macho characteristics" helped him in his sexual conquests: "women love me because I haven't had to develop so many of those unpleasant male traits." But, according to Ganapati Durgadas [7] in Kathleen LeBesco's *Revolting Bodies*, fat feminizes men in a potentially dangerous manner. "The roundness and softness of fat men confirms their 'womanishness' ... their relative male status is revoked." Even among gay and bisexual men, fat can have a feminizing effect. Fat men are "less like men and more like women. Fleshy bulk or stoutness in females implies inappropriate strength or toughness. In males, it represents womanlike weakness or physical impressionability." However, among gay men, there is a separate sexualization of fatness, or "heft," which has become fetishized. Aside from gay or straight men who appear feminized by their obesity, another subgroup is the large, hirsute Bear; "a large or husky body, heavy body hair, a lumbering gait, an epicurean appetite, an attitude of imperturbability, a contented self-acceptance of his own masculinity." According to the Bear Handbook, some men will use the epithet "Bear" to justify overeating, thereby putting their health at risk, by prioritizing their sexuality.

Conclusion

An academic study in 2008 [8] looked scientifically at the link between size and sexuality, dampening speculation on the differences in sexuality between lean and obese individuals, discovering that BMI was not significantly associated with sexual orientation, age at first intercourse, frequency of heterosexual intercourse, and the number of lifetime or current male partners. Overweight women and obese women were more likely to report ever having sexual intercourse with a man, but otherwise, sexual behavior differed little between women of different BMIs. Kate Harding of "Shapely Prose: Home of the Mordantly Obese" website explains, "The world is not full of Attractive People and Unattractive People. It's full of people who are attractive to some and not to others" [9].

References

1. Duke University, 2004.
2. http://www.thefirstpost.co.uk/1953,news-comment,news-politics.
3. http://blogs.telegraph.co.uk/news/peterfoster/9577007/When_will_Mao_enter_the_props_cupboard_of_Chinese_history/.
4. http://www.jimgoad.net/pdf/sex/feeders.pdf. 11.12.2009
5. http://www.naafaonline.com/dev2/
6. http://www.naafaonline.com/dev2//about/Policies/FEEDERISM.pdf. 11.12.2009
7. LeBesco K. Revolting bodies. Amherst: University of Massachusetts Press; 2004.
8. Kaneshiro B, Jensen JT, Carlson NE, Harvey SM, Nichols MD, Edelman AB. Body mass index and sexual behavior. Obstet Gynecol. 2008;112(3):586–92.
9. http://kateharding.net/.

Chapter 7
Fat on Display

David W. Haslam

Oh they are fat, so terribly, terribly, terrifically fat [1].

Beth Ditto is a self-proclaimed "fat feminist lesbian from Arkansas" [2]—confident, attractive, and a successful punk star, recently voted "The Coolest Person on the Planet." A "glamorous and sexy" style icon, she is obsessed by sex. "I think about sex constantly—if you don't think about it constantly, you haven't had really good sex" [3]. She is morbidly obese. Sunday Times journalist Giles Hattersley became excited on having his head "planted between her astonishing bosoms": "Wowzers! … Her body is mesmeric. Rolls and folds topped with an adorable heart-shaped face" [4]. Popular reaction to her size was revealed by the back-handed compliment of her appearance in Virgin's Top Ten Unlikeliest Sex Symbols [5]. Obesity is more than ever on display, on our streets, in restaurants, and in schools; bulging midriffs under skimpy T-shirts are commonplace and not considered unusual. This chapter considers the display of fat.

Until 2009 the oldest known piece of figurative art on Earth was a 25,000-year-old, beautifully sculpted representation of an obese woman, Venus of Willendorf. She is portrayed to anatomical perfection with obese belly; hands resting on

D.W. Haslam, MBBS, DGM
Doctor's Surgery, Watton Place Clinic,
60 High Street, Watton at Stone, SG143SY, UK
e-mail: dwhaslam@aol.com

D.W. Haslam et al. (eds.), *Controversies in Obesity*,
DOI 10.1007/978-1-4471-2834-2_7,
© Springer-Verlag London 2014

breasts, just big enough to rest in the palm of the hand. Her purpose is open to conjecture; some say she is a fertility symbol, others already pregnant, although the Austrian archaeologists who discovered her gave her the moniker "Venus" in a cruel display of sarcasm. However, in 2009 *Nature* magazine presented a statuette 10,000 years older than Venus of Willendorf, from Germany, carved from mammoth ivory— once again, a naked, obese woman. University of Cambridge anthropologist Paul Mellars explained: "If there's one conclusion you want to draw from this, it's that an obsession with sex goes back at least 35,000 years … if humans hadn't been largely obsessed with sex they wouldn't have survived for the first 2 million years." The French, typically, described Venuses as *"prototypes paléolithiques de la playgirl du mois."*

A more recent Venus displayed a different type of obesity. The "Hottentot Venus," Saartjie Baartman, was a young Khoisan woman from the Gamtoos River region of Africa who displayed steatopygia—exaggerated, obese, protruding buttocks and elongated labia—which identified her profound ethnic differences, which perplexed, fascinated, and horrified Europeans in the early nineteenth century. Displayed throughout Europe in life and as anatomical specimens after her death at 35, Saartjie's buttocks represented evidence of the contemporary belief of African women's propensity to excess and deviant sexuality [6]. The display of fat is deeply entrenched in history and many different cultures. The Jewesses of Tunis were fattened for the benefit of men "when scarcely ten years old … by confinement in narrow, dark rooms, where they are fed on farinaceous foods and the flesh of young puppies until they are almost a shapeless mass of fat" [7]. In Mauritania, many girls are force-fed at puberty to make them more alluring to men and thus enhance their marriage prospects. In Japan, sumo wrestlers are both cultural and sexual icons. They are known for their fornicating as much as their eating; a top-ranked sumo wrestler can allegedly point to any women they want for sex [8], and reports of sex orgies have caused scandal. Indian Bollywood actresses are routinely airbrushed on posters to display additional curves to add to their appeal.

One of the earliest known examples of an obese person being commercially displayed was a Welshman known only as G. Hopkins, displayed at a London Fair, possibly the Bartholomew

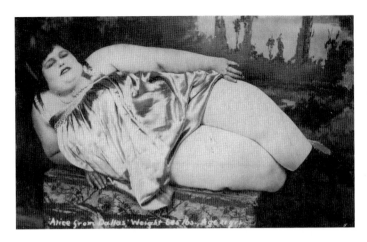

FIGURE 7.1 Circus Fat Lady Alice Wade, "Alice from Dallas"

Fair, in a cart pulled by four teams of oxen, weighing 980 lb, and displayed alongside some prize hogs. Legend has it that after a particularly large meal, he toppled, reaching for a last morsel, and landed on a nursing sow and her piglets, killing them all. The fair was made famous by playwright Ben Jonson in 1631 in *Bartholomew Fayre* featuring the grossly obese Ursula, the pig-woman who deals in "various kinds of flesh" and is "belly, womb, gaping mouth, udder, the source and object of praise and abuse." Above all, like the giant hog displayed at the fair, she is excessive. Like the pigs that she roasts, her element is grease: she is a "walking sow of tallow" and "a whole shire of butter," and her language is "greasier than her pigs." She is the celebrant of the open orifice [9].

Until recently obesity was routinely displayed at circus and carnival sideshows: exhibits such as the tattooed lady and fat ladies would use their unique qualities as excuses to show more flesh than normal. Patrons were allowed to touch their arms and legs before pulling the whiskers of Bearded Ladies. It was deeply arousing to Victorians to touch a strange woman in a quasi-legitimate, respectable setting, and a tantalizing and disturbing sight for the other spectators. A wondrously titillating dialectic emerged, in which performers were perceived as alluring as well as repulsive. A glance at circus Fat Lady Alice Wade, "Alice from Dallas," (Fig. 7.1)

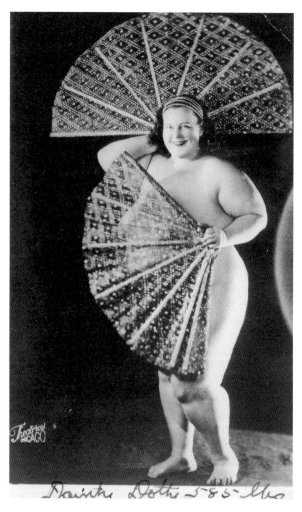

FIGURE 7.2 Dainty Dotty

doesn't reveal a shrinking violet, more an open invitation. In later, more permissive eras, performers such as Dainty Dotty (Fig. 7.2) and Miss Baby Dumpling were overtly provocative, appearing naked behind fans, "400 lbs of fun."

Helen Melon, aka actress Katy Dierlam, performed in the 1990s, recreating the appeal of the Carnival Midway at New York's Coney Island. Charismatic and self-confident, she relentlessly displayed sexuality. Her stage name has sexual connotations, and opening routine involves touching her breasts and shimmying: "Take a good long look!" Her husband Ned Sonntag, a Fat Admirer and illustrator, considers that truly fat women have breast-like areas all over their body, like the ancient fertility goddess Astarte, covered with breasts [10].

Helen Melon explains the basis of the eroticism of the fat woman; "the memory of having been cuddled against the buxom breast of a warm, soft Giantess, whose bulk, to our 8 lb, 21 inch infant selves—must have seemed as mountainous as any 600-lb Fat Lady to our adult selves." Later, saucy seaside postcards including rotund sexually stereotypical women with downtrodden husbands, coupled with juvenile double entendres, became popular.

Fat men also appeared in the side shows but also on private display. The most famous of all—Daniel Lambert— was "viewed" by royalty and aristocracy at his premises in Piccadilly before he died in 1809 at age 34. Later, individuals like Robert Earl Hughes (Fig. 7.3) gained prominence through the media. Although circus sideshows have thankfully disappeared, the sensationalism remains in voyeuristic television programs such as Half Ton Man, which followed the weight-loss attempts of Patrick Deuel, who weighed 510 kg at his peak but lost 318 kg following bariatric surgery.

Pornography involving morbidly obese women—but not men—is common. Videos such as Chunky Chicks and Scale Bustin' Bimbos are commonplace, showing women posing provocatively, rather than indulging in explicit sexual behavior. The stomach and breasts are usually the focus rather than genitalia. Photo shoots often involve erotic and exuberant use of food, typically ice cream, clotted cream, syrup, or spaghetti. Food entering the mouth is a surrogate for sexual penetration. Men who access fat partners or pornography

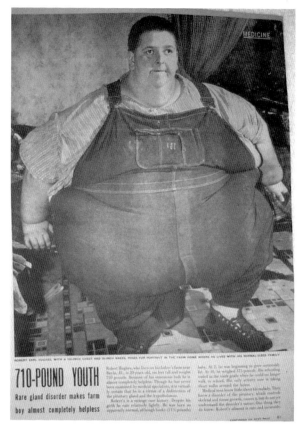

FIGURE 7.3 Robert Earl Hughes

have been labelled Chubby Chasers. "The woman he ended up marrying made him look like a sock puppet when the two were cuddling together" [11].

UK daytime television star Vanessa Feltz describes the attraction between average-sized men and obese women as the only genuine display of true affection: "Men who genuinely love women fantasize about being smothered in sofa-sized breasts and pillowed in marshmallow thighs. Pert is OK but pneumatic is heaven. Not for them the bite-sized morsel. They revel in handfuls, fistfuls, and armfuls of lusty lady" [12].

Fat acceptance such as Feltz's has the problem that high cardiovascular and metabolic disease risk and premature mortality must also be accepted. It is certainly possible to be fat and fit, but this is a common argument used in their defense by fat, blatantly unfit individuals. Today, despite the obesity epidemic, there is an obsession with thinness, compared to Renaissance values, whereby beauty was ascribed to Rubenesque curves. In the 1950s Marilyn Monroe and Jane Russell were pinups, whereas today they would be plump, compared to Kate Moss or Luisel Ramos, whose death during Uruguay's fashion week, after days of starvation, sparked the "size zero" controversy. A review of *Vogue* and *Ladies' Home Journal* from 1901 to 1980 revealed that breast-to-waist ratio among models ranged from 2:0 in 1910 to 1:1 in 1925, 1:5 in 1950, and 1:25 in 1981.

Cass Elliott, aka Mama Cass, of the Mamas and Papas was similarly iconic to Beth Ditto, admired and accepted as an obese role model, until she succumbed to heart failure due to fatty myocardial infiltration, during a solo tour to London on 29 July 1974, age only 32. Big Punisher, one of the first major Rap stars, was regarded as a wealthy and successful family man. He died of a heart attack in 2000 at only 28, weighing 698 lb. Even The King, the ultimate sex symbol, Elvis Presley, paid for a lifestyle of eating Denver Fools Gold Loaf and squirrels fried in butter, dying of a presumed heart attack in Memphis on August 16, 1977, aged 42, as a direct result of his obesity. Fat acceptance and obesity as a lifestyle choice are arguably acceptable, as long as the genuine health risks are acknowledged and tackled. Fat is on display wherever we look; the shameful voyeurism of morbid obesity in the media is making an unwelcome recent comeback.

References

1. Thomson RG. Freakery: cultural spectacles of the extraordinary body. New York: New York University Press; 1996. p. 127–30.
2. http://www.dailymail.co.uk/tvshowbiz/article-1145131/15-stone-Beth-Ditto-launches-Love-magazine-nude-shoot.html.

3. http://www.monstersandcritics.com/people/news/article_1334466.php/Beth_Dittos_24-hour_sex_wish#ixzz0YoiMi5PO.

4. http://women.timesonline.co.uk/tol/life_and_style/women/fashion/article6462773.ece.

5. http://www.virginmedia.com/music/pictures/toptens/unlikely-sex-symbols.php.

6. Mendible M. Bananas to buttocks: the Latina body in popular film and culture. Austin: University of Texas Press; 2007.

7. Gould GM, Pyle W. Anomalies and curiosities of medicine. Philadelphia: WB Saunders; 1901. p. 356.

8. http://news.3yen.com/2005-08-11/do-sumo-enjoy-sex/.

9. Stallybrass P, Allon White A. The politics and poetics of transgression. Ithaca: Cornell University Press; 1986. p. 62–5.

10. http://cache.zoominfo.com/CachedPage/?archive_id=0&page_id=330921100&page_url=%2f%2fwww.deviantdesires.com%2fmap%2ffas.html&page_last_updated=12%2f10%2f2007+8%3a52%3a31+PM&firstName=Conrad&lastName=Blickenstorfer.

11. http://boards.askmen.com/showthread.php?109544-Chubby-chasers. Accessed 4 June 2013.

12. Feltz V. Who says fat isn't sexy?. Revolting Bodies. http://books.google.co.uk/books?id=W7Wz4EKksUcC&pg=PA45&lpg=PA45&dq=vanessa+feltz+%22sofa-sized+breasts%22&source=bl&ots=-kdMzqCSIw&sig=TcH2M5aPxn1jeGZrDJU5e4yZk0E&hl=en&sa=X&ei=UjR1UeL-CeyV0QWf3YGIBw&sqi=2&ved=0CDEQ6AEwAA#v=onepage&q=vanessa%20feltz%20%22sofa-sized%20breasts%22&f=false.

Part III
Causes

Chapter 8
The Emerging Paradigm Shift in Understanding the Causes of Obesity

Shamil A. Chandaria

The Folk Theory of Obesity

The "Folk Theory of Obesity" is the term used here to describe the conventional view that captures the commonsense understanding that the *cause* of obesity is long-term imbalance between energy intake and energy expenditure. The supposed rock-solid justification of this hypothesis is the first law of thermodynamics, effectively the law of conservation of energy (E) applied to a biological system over a certain time period:

$$E_{\text{stored}} = E_{\text{intake}} - E_{\text{expenditure}}$$

A further assumption normally made is that weight gain/loss over the period is approximately proportional to the energy stored. If most of the weight gain/loss is assumed to be fat mass, then the constant of proportionality is approximately 7,500 kCal per kg. Expressing this as an equation, we have for a specified time period

$$\text{Weight}_{\text{gain(kg)}} = \frac{E_{\text{IN(kCal)}} - E_{\text{OUT(kCal)}}}{7,500 \text{kCal} / \text{kg}}$$

S.A. Chandaria, PhD
National Obesity Forum, 76 Harley Street,
London, W1G 7HH, UK
e-mail: schandaria@ampcap.com

D.W. Haslam et al. (eds.), *Controversies in Obesity*,
DOI 10.1007/978-1-4471-2834-2_8,
© Springer-Verlag London 2014

So far so good, the above equation ("energy imbalance equation") is broadly correct, but it is not the various approximations assumed in its derivation that will be critiqued here. There is one final step in the justification of the Folk Theory of Obesity, and this is the one to watch: Energy intake (E_{IN}) and energy expenditure (E_{OUT}) are exogenous variables, and weight gain is a fully endogenous variable. Roughly this could also be stated as energy intake (E_{IN}) and energy expenditure (E_{OUT}) are independent variables, and weight gain is a fully dependent variable. This implies that the right-hand side of the energy imbalance equation (calories in–calories out) *causes* the left-hand side (weight gain). But there is no such causality embedded into the first law of thermodynamics. There is no theoretical reason why causality may not operate in the reverse direction; that is, weight gain may, via homeostatic mechanisms, regulate energy intake and energy expenditure. The next section will look at epidemiological data that show that there must be some such homeostatic mechanisms. The sections thereafter will explore the details of these mechanisms and show that when such mechanisms become dysfunctional, they can result in the development of obesity.

A Challenge to the Folk Theory of Obesity from Epidemiological Data

Epidemiological data show that over a 10-year period the average change in a person's weight is less than about 10 kg over the decade and the median person's weight change is closer to 5 kg over the decade [1–4]. A calculation can be done to examine how tightly on average we have to regulate our calorie balance over a decade to keep our weight change to less than 10 kg.

1. As already noted, 1 kg is equivalent to about 7,500 kCal.
2. So 10 kg is equivalent to $10 \times 7,500$ kCal which is 75,000 kCal.
3. Assuming a person consumes on average 2,500 kCal/day.
4. Then over 10 years (3,650 days) the person consumes $3,650 \times 2,500$ kCal which is 9,125,000 kCal/decade.

5. So the error in perfect energy balance over a decade is 75,000/9,125,000, which is an error of 0.82 %.
6. Or expressed another way we are able to keep calories consumed balanced with calorie expenditure with an accuracy of 99.18 %.
7. Or expressed another way the average error in balancing our energy inflow vs. our energy expenditure on a daily basis is 0.82 % × 2,500 kCal/day, which is 21 kCal day – a tablespoon of food.

For the Folk Theory of Obesity to hold, one would have to have to assume that we can exogenously or independently balance our energy consumption and our energy expenditure to be within 99 % of each other. This is an unreasonable assumption. There must be some homeostatic mechanism or mechanisms that influence the consumption of calories and the body's energy expenditure making these variables partly endogenous and influenced by weight gain. Specifically, what this numerical exercise has alluded to is the idea that when the weight of a person fluctuates, say increases, there must be some negative feedback mechanisms to reduce calorie intake and/or increase calorie expenditure (and vice versa for weight loss). Indeed, there are such mechanisms and a very direct one was discovered in 1994 and involves the hormone leptin.

Homeostatic Mechanisms

Leptin is a hormone that is released by adipocytes, and its plasma concentration is positively correlated with total fat mass [5–7]. Leptin activates specific receptors in the brain located mostly in the arcuate nucleus of the hypothalamus, thereby giving the brain a direct signal of the amount of adiposity in the body. This leptin signal to the hypothalamus then regulates calorie intake, by increasing satiety and reducing appetite, and calorie expenditure by increasing adaptive thermogenesis (surplus heat production over and above that required for basal metabolism and physical activity) [8].

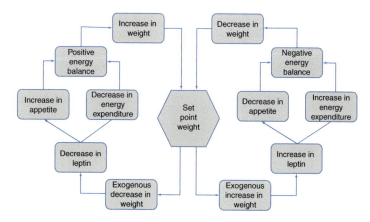

FIGURE 8.1 A mechanistic basis for the set point theory of weight

So, for example, if a person has an exogenous weight gain, increased adiposity will lead to increased leptin levels, and this signal will reduce appetite, increase satiety, and increase energy expenditure. This will then tend to create a negative energy balance and thus lead to weight loss. Similarly, an exogenous weight loss will depress leptin levels and will increase appetite, reduce satiety, and decrease energy expenditure.

If this leptin mechanism works correctly, a reverse causality has been introduced into the energy imbalance equation (from the LHS to the RHS) and so the Folk Theory of Obesity loses its theoretical justification. We also have a mechanistic basis for the "set point theory of weight," the view that the body has a normal weight that it defends and reverts to after deviations from that weight. Figure 8.1 illustrates set point mechanism.

A Mechanistic Basis for the Set Point Theory of Weight

Since the discovery of leptin, numerous other hormonal and neural signals that directly affect energy balance have been discovered. One important class of signals is the *gut peptides*

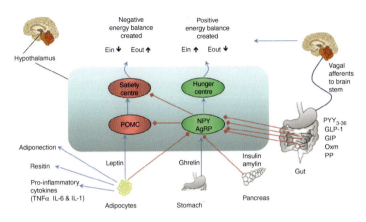

FIGURE 8.2 Homeostatic signals that regulate energy balance

that are released when nutrients come into contact with the walls of the gut. These peptide hormonal signals are an indication of an energy inflow into the body and act on the hypothalamus to cause a reduction in appetite and increase energy expenditure. This is a short-term homeostatic signal. Examples of these signals include peptide YY (PYY), glucagon-like peptide-1 (GLP-1), glucose-dependent insulinotropic polypeptide (GIP), and oxyntomodulin. Each type of peptide is released differentially depending on the type of calories and the position in the gut, thus conveying rich informational signals to the brain. *Insulin* and *amylin*, hormones released by the pancreas, are sensed by the hypothalamus and induce appetite reduction and energy expenditure. Again this is a homeostatic signal since high levels of these hormones normally indicate a high level of energy availability in the blood, namely, glucose. Figure 8.2 shows these and other homeostatic signals.

Metabolic Dysfunction: The Proximate Causes of Obesity

So with all these wonderful homeostatic mechanisms, one might ask, why is there any obesity at all? It's a good question that hasn't yet got a fully integrative answer. But we have started to identify some of the factors that are involved. These factors either directly disrupt the homeostatic mechanisms described above or disrupt parts of the body's metabolism that indirectly disrupts the energy homeostasis. It's worth mentioning a few of these "metabolic disruptors," but it should be noted that the causal interactions between these disruptors are not yet fully understood.

Soon after the discovery of leptin, it emerged that while obese people had higher plasma leptin levels (as expected since they had more fat mass), this leptin signal was not able to reduce appetite and increase thermogenesis. Somehow, somewhere in the brain there was a blunting of this signal. This has been termed "leptin resistance." Understanding the causes of leptin resistance is one of the holy grails of obesity research. It isn't known whether leptin resistance is a cause or a result of obesity. It could even be that some other metabolic disruptor, such as insulin resistance, influences leptin resistance. But what is known is that in obese individuals a major homeostatic mechanism is disrupted.

Another class of metabolic disruption is *gut peptide dysfunction*. Obese individuals tend to have low secretions of GLP-1 and PYY following meal ingestion [9]. Changes in gut architecture following bariatric surgery can increase these secretions dramatically, and it is thought that this is a major mechanism for the success of these operations in reducing obesity, effectively reinstituting or strengthening broken homeostatic mechanisms.

Insulin resistance is probably the most important metabolic disruptor and is at the heart of the "metabolic syndrome" – a cluster of correlated disorders that include central obesity, dyslipidemia, hypertension, and impaired fasting glucose. The effects of insulin resistance and associated elevated insulin levels on the liver, skeletal muscle, adipose tissue, and the brain are complex and interacting and disrupt many energy and fuel partitioning systems in the body. For example, chronically elevated insulin levels prevent triglycerides from being released from fat cells and separately promote the synthesis of fatty acids in the liver. Together this effectively creates one-way traffic, shunting energy into fat storage with little regard to the energy requirements of the body.

Other metabolic disruptors might include chronic stress reactions/HPA axis dysfunction, low-grade inflammation, gut flora disruption, androgen balance disruption, and adipokine dysfunction.

These metabolic disruptors may interact with one another in a web of interactions, effectively creating a vicious cycle. It is this vicious cycle that is the etiology of obesity. So metabolic disruptors such as leptin resistance, gut peptide dysfunction, insulin resistance, HPA axis dysfunction, low-grade inflammation gut flora ecosystem disruption, and adipokine dysfunction operate together (in a web of associations the details of which are still to be worked out) to *cause* a disruption in the fine energy homeostasis that characterizes a healthy human body. The result is obesity.

Genetics, Epigenetics, and Environment: The Underlying Causes of Obesity

So far, the *proximate causes* of obesity – metabolic disruptors at the biochemical and mechanistic level – have been discussed. But what are the *underlying causes* that ultimately create these metabolic dysfunctions themselves? There are many hypotheses, but since the objective here is to understand the emerging paradigm, the basic structure – leaving open the final details whatever they may turn out to be – will be sketched.

Twins studies show that genes strongly influence the individual variation in obesity. Data from 25,000 twin pairs show that the correlation between the BMI of monozygotic twins (who share the same genes and the same environment) is 0.74, but the correlation is 0.32 between dizygotic twins (who share the same environment but only some of the genes) [10]. But while genetic factors are clearly important in the development of obesity, they cannot explain the rising tide of obesity in

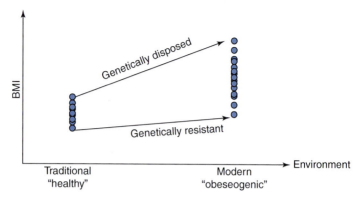

FIGURE 8.3 A stylized model for the interaction of genes and the environment

recent decades – the gene pool cannot have changed over such a short time period. Our environment on the other hand has changed significantly over this period. Might there be environmental factors that cause metabolic dysfunction in those who have a genetic disposition to be so affected by such factors? These putative factors are termed "obesogenic" environmental factors. Many such factors have been proposed: sedentary lifestyle, processed foods, refined carbohydrates, high sugar consumption, easy access to food, larger portion sizes, more stressful lives, and so forth. Figure 8.3 shows a stylized model for the interaction of genes and the environment. Those in a population that are genetically disposed to obesity are the ones who increase their BMI most when impacted by an obesogenic environment.

One important complication in this story is that it is not just our inherited genes that predispose us to metabolic dysfunction, but epigenetic factors induced in early environment can have a similar effect. Early environmental factors such as impaired maternal blood sugar control during pregnancy, maternal stress, low birth weight, and formula milk rather than breast feeding may cause changes to the genome, such as DNA methylation, which permanently affect gene expression [11]. These changes may increase the risk of developing

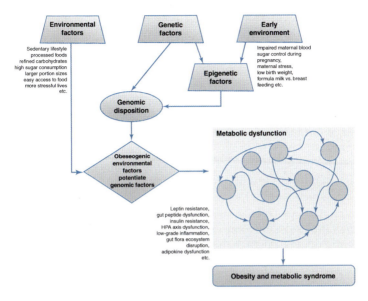

FIGURE 8.4 Schematic of the new emerging paradigm of the causes of obesity

metabolic dysfunction later in life (especially in the face of later obesogenic environmental factors) and so lead to obesity. Figure 8.4 is a schematic that summarizes the emerging paradigm of the causes of obesity.

Implications of the Emerging Paradigm

The Folk Theory paradigm of obesity has clear and *apparently* logical intervention strategies to combat obesity: if obesity is caused by taking in more calories than are being burnt over the long term, then to combat obesity a person should actively reduce their calorie intake and purposefully increase physical activity to burn more calories. Of course, it should now be understood that this logic is flawed because energy intake and energy expenditure are not exogenous variables. They are partly regulated and influenced by the hypothalamus. If we move towards the view that obesity is better understood as a metabolic and hormonal disorder, then interventional strategies should be based on improving the underlying metabolic and hormonal dysfunction in the face of an obesogenic environment.

Intervention strategies to combat obesity are best understood as not acting directly on long-term energy balance but indirectly influencing obesity by acting through the metabolism. For example, exercise may be an important intervention not simply because it burns calories but because it can improve insulin sensitivity and help to normalize stress hormones. Another example might be that reducing the consumption of refined carbohydrates might help to improve metabolic dysfunction caused by high levels of insulin. Or antioxidants might help to improve some other aspect of metabolic disruption.

The emerging paradigm sees the causes of obesity as a metabolic and hormonal dysfunction and thus moves the basis of interventional strategies from trying to influence human agency – battling gluttony and sloth – to trying to influence human biology. This is an important step.

References

1. Lewis CE, Jacobs Jr DR, McCreath H, Kiefe CI, Schreiner PJ, Smith DE, Williams OD. Weight gain continues in the 1990s: 10-year trends in weight and overweight from the CARDIA study. Coronary Artery Risk Development in Young Adults. Am J Epidemiol. 2000;151(12):1172–81.
2. http://www.alswh.org.au/Reports/Achievements/achievements-weight.pdf. Australian Longitudinal Study on Women's Health. Research highlights – the first decade: Australian women and their weight – a growing problem. 2005. http://www.newcastle.edu.au/centre/wha/Reports/achievements_reports.html.
3. Resnick HE, Valsania P, Halter JB, Lin X. Relation of weight gain and weight loss on subsequent diabetes risk in overweight adults. J Epidemiol Community Health. 2000;54:596–602.
4. Resnicka HE, Valsaniab P, Halterc JB, Lind XJ. Relation of weight gain and weight loss on subsequent diabetes risk in overweight adults. J Epidemiol Community Health. 2000;54:596–602.

5. Zhang Y, Proenca R, Maffei M, Barone M, Leopold L, Friedman JM. Positional cloning of the mouse obese gene and its human homologue. Nature. 1994;372:425–32.

6. Maffei M, Halaas J, Ravussin E, Pratley RE, Lee GH, Zhang Y, et al. Leptin levels in human and rodent: measurement of plasma leptin and ob RNA in obese and weight-reduced subjects. Nat Med. 1995;1:1155–61.

7. Considine RV, Sinha MK, Heiman ML, Kriauciunas A, Stephens TW, Nyce MR, et al. Serum immunoreactive-leptin concentrations in normal-weight and obese humans. N Engl J Med. 1996;334:292–5.

8. Spiegelman BM, Flier JS. Obesity and the regulation of energy balance. Cell. 2001;104:531–43.

9. Morínigo R, Moizé V, Musri M, Lacy AM, Navarro S, Marín JL, et al. Glucagon-like peptide-1, peptide YY, hunger, and satiety after gastric bypass surgery in morbidly obese subjects. J Clin Endocrinol Metab. 2006;91(5):1735–40.

10. Maes HH, Neale MC, Eaves LJ. Genetic and environmental factors in relative body weight and human adiposity. Behav Genet. 1997;27:325–51.

11. Gluckman PD, Hanson MA. Developmental and epigenetic pathways to obesity: an evolutionary-developmental perspective. Int J Obes. 2008;32:S62–71.

Chapter 9
Adenoviruses and Obesity

Richard L. Atkinson

A past president of The Obesity Society (TOS) who shall go unnamed said to a reporter, "Obesity is a very complex disease that results from eating too much." This illustrates the simplistic nature by which even obesity experts approach the etiology of obesity. A TOS committee charged with writing a white paper regarding whether obesity is a "disease" concluded that technically it is not a disease, but TOS would consider it one [1]. Given this background, the concept that a virus causes some cases of obesity has met with stiff resistance from both scientists and the lay public. The implications of a viral etiology of obesity have major ramifications, both socially and economically. An infectious etiology of obesity may be prevented with a suitable vaccine, and the current discrimination against obesity would have to be reexamined. This chapter will give the evidence that adenovirus 36 (Adv36) causes obesity in animals and humans, perhaps accounting for a major portion of the worldwide epidemic of obesity that has occurred since 1980.

Starting about 1980 the prevalence of obesity began to rise worldwide, in both developed and undeveloped countries [2]. Obesity doubled in adults and tripled in children in the USA,

R.L. Atkinson, MD
Department of Pathology, Virginia Commonwealth University,
Obetech Obesity Research Center, Obetech, LLC,
800 East Leigh St., Richmond, VA 23111, USA
e-mail: ratkinson2@vcu.edu

D.W. Haslam et al. (eds.), *Controversies in Obesity*,
DOI 10.1007/978-1-4471-2834-2_9,
© Springer-Verlag London 2014

with similar or even greater rises in other countries [2–12]. The global nature of this rise argues against simple changes in diet, lifestyle, and physical activity and suggests a ubiquitous environmental factor might be responsible. While some type of industrial pollutant causing obesity is possible, an infectious agent would be the most plausible cause of the epidemic. Adv36 was first isolated in 1978 [13], about the same time as the appearance of an avian adenovirus (SMAM-1) in chickens in India that was shown to be responsible for an accelerated death rate in commercial chicken flocks and obesity in infected chickens [14]. SMAM-1 decreases immune function in chickens, leading to a somewhat increased death rate and accumulation of excess fat, particularly visceral fat [14]. About 20 % of obese patients in a study in India had antibodies to this virus and were significantly heavier than uninfected patients [15]. We postulated that this chicken virus mutated to be able to infect humans and cause obesity [15, 16].

Adv36 is a human adenovirus that causes a mild upper respiratory illness with experimental infection in animals [16–21]. Experimental infection of chickens, mice, rats, and monkeys with Adv36 causes obesity in 60–100 % (100 % of monkeys) with an increase in adipose tissue of 50–150 % depending on animal and experiment [16–21]. Food intake is not increased, and activity levels do not appear increased compared to uninfected controls [16, 17, 19, 20]. The infection is spread between animals by respiratory droplets and likely in feces [16, 17, 20]. The infection is highly contagious, and uninfected chickens in the same cage with infected chickens quickly developed infection and became obese [17, 20]. Transfusion of 200 μL of blood from infected chickens caused infection and obesity in recipient chickens [17]. Mice appear to be infectious for 4–8 weeks after experimental infection [20], and live virus could be grown from monkeys up to 2 months after infection [18]. Adv36 DNA could be recovered from tissues 7 months after the initial infection, long after live virus could not be isolated [18]. Experimental infection of animals results in improved glucose transport, lower serum insulin levels, and lower levels of serum cholesterol and triglycerides [16–19].

Experimental infection in humans would not be ethical, but past infection may be determined by evaluation of serum for antibodies to Adv36. Adv36 is different from almost all other human adenoviruses in that antibodies to Adv36 do not neutralize other adenoviruses in tissue culture and antibodies to other adenoviruses do not neutralize Adv36 [13]. Therefore, presence of Adv36 antibodies is evidence of prior infection. Adv36 antibodies may be detected by serum neutralization assay [22–31] or by ELISA assay [32]. Infection also may be detected by assay of Adv36 DNA in tissues, particularly adipose tissue using polymerase chain reaction (PCR) methods [18, 33]. The first assessment of prevalence of Adv36 infection in humans showed that 30 % of obese adults and 11 % of nonobese adults had Adv36 antibodies and infected individuals were significantly heavier than uninfected [22]. Paradoxically, serum cholesterol and triglycerides were lower in infected individuals [22], similar to the changes in experimentally infected animals [16–19]. Multiple studies have demonstrated that the prevalence of Adv36 infection averages about 30 % in obese adults and children, with a range of 6–65 % [22–32]. Most studies in adults show a correlation of body weight or fat to Adv36 infection, but two studies do not [25, 26]. A potential problem in interpreting studies in adults is the loss of antibodies over time after the initial infection, resulting in serum assays that are negative. Since the time from the initial infection is likely to be shorter, we would expect studies in children to show a closer association of Adv36 status and obesity. Indeed, this is the case, with all five studies in children having some type of correlation of Adv36 status with obesity [28–32]. Combining all published studies in children reveals a total of 983 children with 28 % of obese children and 17 % of nonobese children being Adv36 positive [28–32].

The mechanisms of Adv36 obesity are due to the early gene 4, open reading frame 1 (E4orf1) of Adv36 [34, 35]. Blocking the E4orf1 gene blocks the obesity effect, and transfecting this gene into a lentivirus confers the obesity effect to the lentivirus [34, 35]. With infection there are changes in a wide variety of biochemical pathways resulting in an increase of glucose receptors in the cell membrane due to stimulation of the Ras pathway and an increase in fatty acid synthase (FAS) mRNA and protein [34–46]. This increased FAS converts glucose to fatty acids in several types of cells infected with Adv36 [34–46]. The PPAR-gamma pathway is stimulated as well, resulting in differentiation of adult stem cells in adipose tissue [36, 37, 40]. Therefore, fat pads of infected animals versus uninfected animals showed both hypertrophy and hyperplasia [16, 37, 40].

In summary, Adv36 has been shown definitively to cause obesity in multiple animal species and is strongly associated with obesity in humans. About 30 % of obese adults and children are positive, suggesting that if the hypothesis is correct that Adv36 mutated from an animal virus around 1980, it is responsible for a major portion of the worldwide epidemic of obesity. A virus-induced etiology of obesity requires that policies of government and insurance companies toward obesity must change and perhaps may help correct the prejudice that obesity is simply a lack of willpower. It raises hope that a vaccine to prevent Adv36 obesity may have a large impact on the prevalence of obesity throughout the world.

Conflict of Interest The author is the owner of Obetech, LLC. This small business provides assays for adenoviruses that produce obesity and has multiple patents in the area of virus-induced obesity, diagnostic assays, and vaccines.

References

1. Allison DB, Downey M, Atkinson RL, Billington CJ, Bray GA, Eckel RH, et al. Obesity as a disease: a white paper on evidence and arguments commissioned by the Council of the Obesity Society. Obesity. 2008;16(6):1161–77.
2. WHO. Preventing and managing the global epidemic of obesity: report of a WHO Consultation on Obesity. Geneva, 3–5 June 1997. Geneva: WHO/NUT/NCD98.1; 1998.
3. Ogden CL, Flegal KM, Carroll MD, Johnson CL. Prevalence and trends in overweight among US children and adolescents, 1999–2000. JAMA. 2002;288:1728–32.

4. Ogden CL, Carroll MD, Kit BK, Flegal KM. Prevalence of obesity and trends in body mass index among US children and adolescents, 1999–2010. JAMA. 2012;307(5):483–90; Epub 2012 Jan 17.
5. Flegal KM, Carroll MD, Ogden CL, Johnson CL. Prevalence and trends in obesity among US adults, 1999–2000. JAMA. 2002; 288(14):1723–7.
6. Ogden CL, Carroll MD, Kit BK, Flegal KM. Prevalence of obesity in the United States, 2009–2010. NCHS Data Brief. 2012;82:1–8.
7. Lobstein T, Baur L, Uauy R, IOTF Childhood Obesity Working Group. Obesity in children and young people: a crisis in public health. Obes Rev. 2004;5 Suppl 1:4–85.
8. James PT. Obesity: the worldwide epidemic. Clin Dermatol. 2004;22(4):276–80.
9. Luo J, Hu FB. Time trends of obesity in pre-school children in China from 1989 to 1997. Int J Obes. 2002;26:553–8.
10. Likitmaskul S, Kiattisathavee P, Chaichanwatanakul K, Punnakanta L, Angsusingha K, Tuchinda C. Increasing prevalence of type 2 diabetes mellitus in Thai children and adolescents associated with increasing prevalence of obesity. J Pediatr Endocrinol Metab. 2003;16(1):71–7.
11. Yoo S, Lee SY, Kim KN, Sung E. Obesity in Korean pre-adolescent school children: comparison of various anthropometric measurements based on bioelectrical impedance analysis. Int J Obes (Lond). 2006;30(7):1086–90.
12. Kim HM, Park J, Kim HS, Kim DH, Park SH. Obesity and cardiovascular risk factors in Korean children and adolescents aged 10–18 years from the Korean National Health and Nutrition Examination Survey, 1998 and 2001. Am J Epidemiol. 2006;164(8): 787–93.
13. Wigand R, Gelderblom H, Wadell G. New human adenovirus (candidate adenovirus 36), a novel member of subgroup D. Arch Virol. 1980;64:225–33.
14. Dhurandhar NV, Kulkarni PR, Ajinkya SM, Sherikar AA. Effect of adenovirus infection on adiposity in chickens. Vet Microbiol. 1992;31:101–7.
15. Dhurandhar NV, Kulkarni PR, Ajinkya SM, Sherikar AA, Atkinson RL. Association of adenovirus infection with human obesity. Obes Res. 1997;5(5):464–9.
16. Dhurandhar NV, Israel BA, Kolesar JM, Cook ME, Atkinson RL. Increased adiposity in animals due to a human virus. Int J Obes. 2000;24:989–96.
17. Dhurandhar NV, Israel BA, Kolesar JM, Mayhew G, Cook ME, Atkinson RL. Transmissibility of adenovirus-induced adiposity in a chicken model. Int J Obes Relat Metab Disord. 2001;25:990–6.
18. Dhurandhar NV, Whigham LD, Abbott DH, Schultz-Darken NJ, Israel BA, Bradley SM, et al. Human adenovirus Ad-36 promotes

weight gain in male rhesus and marmoset monkeys. J Nutr. 2002; 132(10):3155–60.

19. Whigham LD, Israel BA, Atkinson RL. Adipogenic potential of multiple human adenoviruses in vivo and in vitro in animals. Am J Physiol Regul Integr Comp Physiol. 2006;290:R190–4.

20. Pasarica M, Shin AC, Yu M, Ou Yang HM, Rathod M, Jen KL, et al. Human adenovirus 36 induces adiposity, increases insulin sensitivity, and alters hypothalamic monoamines in rats. Obesity (Silver Spring). 2006;14(11):1905–13.

21. Na HN, Nam JH. Adenovirus 36 as an obesity agent maintains the obesity state by increasing MCP-1 and inducing inflammation. J Infect Dis. 2012;205(6):914–22; Epub 2012 Jan 24.

22. Atkinson RL, Dhurandhar NV, Allison DB, Bowen RL, Israel BA, Albu JB, et al. Human adenovirus-36 is associated with increased body weight and paradoxical reduction of serum lipids. Int J Obes (Lond). 2005;29(3):281–6.

23. Trovato GM, Castro A, Tonzuso A, Garozzo A, Martines GF, Pirri C, et al. Human obesity relationship with Ad36 adenovirus and insulin resistance. Int J Obes (Lond). 2009;33(12):1402–9.

24. Trovato GM, Martines GF, Garozzo A, Tonzuso A, Timpanaro R, Pirri C, et al. Ad36 adipogenic adenovirus in human non-alcoholic fatty liver disease. Liver Int. 2010;30(2):184–90; Epub 2009 Oct 13.

25. Broderick MP, Hansen CJ, Irvine M, Metzgar D, Campbell K, Baker C, et al. Adenovirus 36 seropositivity is strongly associated with race and gender, but not obesity, among US military personnel. Int J Obes (Lond). 2010;34(2):302–8; Epub 2009 Nov 10.

26. Goossens VJ, deJager SA, Grauls GE, Gielen M, Vlietinck RF, Derom CA, et al. Lack of evidence for the role of human adenovirus-36 in obesity in a European cohort. Obesity (Silver Spring). 2011;19(1):220–1; Epub 2009 Dec 10.

27. Rubicz R, Leach CT, Kraig E, Dhurandhar NV, Grubbs B, Blangero J, et al. Seroprevalence of 13 common pathogens in a rapidly growing U.S. minority population: Mexican Americans from San Antonio, TX. BMC Res Notes. 2011;4(1):433.

28. Atkinson RL, Lee I, Shin HJ, He J. Human adenovirus-36 antibody status is associated with obesity in children. Int J Pediatr Obes. 2010;5(2):157–60; Epub 2009 Jul 1.

29. Na HN, Hong YM, Kim J, Kim HK, Jo I, Nam JH. Association between human adenovirus-36 and lipid disorders in Korean schoolchildren. Int J Obes. 2010;34(1):89–93; Epub 2009 Oct 13.

30. Gabbert C, Donohue M, Arnold J, Schwimmer JB. Adenovirus 36 and obesity in children and adolescents. Pediatrics. 2010;126(4): 721–6.

31. McAllister EJ, Sothern M, Laramie ELM, et al. In children, infection with adenovirus Ad36 is associated with better metabolic profile. Obesity. 2009;17(S2):S239.

32. Almgren M, Atkinson R, He J, Hilding A, Hagman E, Wolk A, et al. Adenovirus-36 is associated with obesity in children and adults in Sweden as determined by rapid ELISA. PLoS One. 2012;7(7):e41652.

33. Salehian B, Forman SJ, Kandeel FR, Bruner DE, He J, Atkinson RL. Adenovirus 36 DNA in adipose tissue of patient with unusual visceral obesity. Emerg Infect Dis. 2010;16(5):850–2.

34. Rogers PM, Fusinski KA, Rathod MA, Loiler SA, Pasarica M, Shaw MK, et al. Human adenovirus Ad-36 induces adipogenesis via its E4 orf-1 gene. Int J Obes. 2008;32(3):397–406; Epub 2007 Nov 6.

35. Dhurandhar EJ, Dubuisson O, Mashtalir N, Krishnapuram R, Hegde V, Dhurandhar NV. E4orf1: a novel ligand that improves glucose disposal in cell culture. PLoS One. 2011;6(8):e23394. doi:10.1371/journal.pone.0023394.

36. Vangipuram SD, Sheele J, Atkinson RL, Holland TC, Dhurandhar NV. A human adenovirus enhances preadipocyte differentiation. Obes Res. 2004;12(5):770–7.

37. Pasarica M, Mashtalir N, McAllister EJ, Kilroy GE, Koska J, Permana P, et al. Adipogenic human adenovirus Ad-36 induces commitment, differentiation, and lipid accumulation in human adipose-derived stem cells. Stem Cells. 2008;26(4):969–78; Epub 2008 Jan 17.

38. Rogers PM, Mashtalir N, Rathod MA, Dubuisson O, Wang Z, Dasuri K, et al. Metabolically favorable remodeling of human adipose tissue by human adenovirus type 36. Diabetes. 2008;57(9):2321–31; Epub 2008 Jul 3.

39. Wang ZQ, Cefalu WT, Zhang XH, Yu Y, Qin J, Son L, et al. Human adenovirus type 36 enhances glucose uptake in diabetic and nondiabetic human skeletal muscle cells independent of insulin signaling. Diabetes. 2008;57(7):1805–13; Epub 2008 Apr 16.

40. Rathod MA, Rogers PM, Vangipuram SD, McAllister EJ, Dhurandhar NV. Adipogenic cascade can be induced without adipogenic media by a human adenovirus. Obesity (Silver Spring). 2009; 17(4):657–64.

41. Wang ZQ, Yu Y, Zhang XH, Floyd EZ, Cefalu WT. Human adenovirus 36 decreases fatty acid oxidation and increases de novo lipogenesis in primary cultured human skeletal muscle cells by promoting Cidec/FSP27 expression. Int J Obes (Lond). 2010;34(9): 1355–64; Epub 2010 May 4.

42. Dubuisson O, Dhurandhar EJ, Krishnapuram R, Kirk-Ballard H, Gupta AK, Hegde V, et al. PPAR{gamma}-independent increase in glucose uptake and adiponectin abundance in fat cells. Endocrinology. 2011;152(10):3648–60.

43. Na HN, Kim H, Nam JH. Novel genes and cellular pathways related to infection with adenovirus-36 as an obesity agent in human mesenchymal stem cells. Int J Obes (Lond). 2011;36(2):195–200.

44. Krishnapuram R, Dhurandhar EJ, Dubuisson O, Kirk-Ballard H, Bajpeyi S, Butte N, et al. Template to improve glycemic control

without reducing adiposity or dietary fat. Am J Physiol Endocrinol Metab. 2011;300(5):E779–89; Epub 2011 Jan 25.

45. Wang ZQ, Yu Y, Zhang XH, Qin J, Floyd E. Gene expression profile in human skeletal muscle cells infected with human adenovirus type 36. J Med Virol. 2012;84(8):1254–66.

46. Krishnapuram R, Kirk-Ballard H, Dhurandhar EJ, Dubuisson O, Messier V, Rabasa-Lhoret R, et al. Insulin receptor-independent upregulation of cellular glucose uptake. Int J Obes (Lond). 2013;37(1):146–53.

Chapter 10
The Role of the Gut Microbiome in Obesity

Kristine H. Allin and Oluf Pedersen

Trillions of microbes colonize the human body cavities and surfaces, and the vast majority of these microbes live in the distal gut (>1 kg in adults) [1]. The "healthy" gut microbiota has multiple functions: for instance, it contributes to energy extraction through fermentation of dietary fibers with production of monosaccharides and short-chain fatty acids, it has tropic functions on mucosa epithelial cells, it educates the immune system and assists in the defense against pathogens, and it contributes to synthesis of amino acids and vitamins essential for humans [2–4]. Initially, the study of the microbiota was limited to culture-based methods. However, it is estimated that as much as 60 % of the human-associated microorganisms, depending on body site, cannot be cultured [5], and new culture-independent approaches such as pyrosequencing of the species-specific bacterial ribosomal RNA gene (16S rRNA), phylogenetic microarrays, and metagenomic shotgun sequencing have recently been applied to characterize the microbial communities from

K.H. Allin, MD, PhD • O. Pedersen, MD, DMSc (✉)
Faculty of Health and Medical Sciences,
The Novo Nordisk Foundation Center for
Basic Metabolic Research, Section of
Metabolic Genetics, University of Copenhagen,
Universitetsparken 1, Copenhagen 2100, Denmark
e-mail: oluf@sund.ku.dk

D.W. Haslam et al. (eds.), *Controversies in Obesity*,
DOI 10.1007/978-1-4471-2834-2_10,
© Springer-Verlag London 2014

multiple sites of the human body (http://www.metahit.eu and http://commonfund.nih.gov/hmp/). In the human distal gut, these approaches have shown that the vast majority of bacteria belong to three phyla: the Gram-negative *Bacteroidetes* and the Gram-positive *Firmicutes* and *Actinobacteria* [4, 6], and a first reference catalogue of the gut microbiome (the set of genes within the gut microbiota) accounts 3.3 million microbial genes as compared to the about 23,000 genes in the human genome [7]. In contrast to the human genome, the human gut microbiome is constantly changing and influenced by a number of factors including dietary habits [8, 9] and use of antibiotics [10] and likely also by individual variations in the human genome.

Recent studies have suggested that alterations in the gut microbiota composition and function (dysbiosis) may be harmful to host health. Accordingly, observational studies in human obesity have demonstrated reduced bacterial diversity, a relative depletion of *Bacteroidetes*, and enrichment in genes involved in carbohydrate and lipid metabolism [11, 12]. These correlative findings raise the important question of whether the altered gut microbiota is a causal factor in the pathogenesis of obesity or whether the gut dysbiosis is merely an innocent bystander. It has been shown that the obesity-associated gut microbiome has an increased capacity to harvest energy from the diet through increased fermentation of carbohydrates resulting in increased amounts of short-chain fatty acids, mainly acetate, butyrate, and propionate [13]. Also, overfeeding of lean volunteers has been shown to result in a rapid change in gut microbiota with an increase in *Firmicutes* and a decrease in *Bacteroidetes*, paralleled by an increased energy harvest [14]. These findings may imply that high-fat diet itself, and not the obese state, may account for changes in the gut microbiota observed in obesity. In addition to influencing the energy harvest, the gut microbiota also appears to affect host obesity by influencing metabolism and inflammation throughout the body at sites distant to the gut. Bacterial endotoxin (lipopolysaccharide [LPS]) is a component of the cell walls of Gram-negative bacteria, and interestingly, a high-fat diet has been shown to induce increased levels of plasma LPS (metabolic endotoxemia), suggesting that altered gut microbiota and increased intestinal permeability may contribute to postprandial inflammation in humans [15]. Furthermore, studies in rodents have shown that the gut microbiota regulates gut epithelial production of circulating fasting-induced adipose factor (Fiaf) (a lipoprotein lipase inhibitor) [16] as well as levels of gut hormones (i.e., GLP-2) [17]. Interestingly, exposure to antibiotics during the first 6 months of human life has been shown to associate with increases in body mass from 10 to 38 months [18]. The wide use of antibiotics administered in low doses in the agricultural industry inspired a study of subtherapeutic antibiotic therapy in a murine model. This study reported increased adiposity in young mice, and accordingly, changes were found in the composition of the gut microbiome and in copies of key genes involved in metabolism of carbohydrates to short-chain fatty acids [19]. Also, colonic short-chain fatty acid levels were increased, and alterations in the regulation of hepatic metabolism of lipids and cholesterol were shown [19].

The most convincing evidence to support a causal role of the gut microbiota in obesity originates from fecal transplantation studies. Thus, transplantation of fecal samples from obese mice to germ-free healthy mice has shown that obesity can be transferred by the microbiota [13, 20]. Recently, a transplantation study of humans with metabolic syndrome reported that transplantation of microbiota from lean donors resulted in increased insulin sensitivity, increased gut microbial diversity, increased levels of butyrate-producing intestinal microbiota, and a decrease in short-chain fatty acids of recipients [21]. The transplantation of feces, however, is likely a rather broad-spectrum treatment approach with potentially serious side effects such as transmission of colorectal cancer cells from donor to recipient. Therefore, administration of prebiotics (nondigestible but fermentable food ingredients that selectively stimulate the growth or activity of one or multiple gut microbes that are beneficial to their human hosts) or probiotics (food supplements that contain living bacteria such as *Bifidobacteria* that address deficiencies in the host microbiota and confer beneficial effects to the host) may be a more desirable approach. Several mechanistic studies in rodents and fewer human studies have indeed shown promising effects on metabolic disturbances, although large prospective randomized controlled trials in humans demonstrating changes in the composition of the gut microbiota after prebiotic or probiotic treatment are lacking [22].

To better understand the link between the gut microbiota and obesity, future studies in individuals with obesity must apply integrative approaches using genomics, metagenomics, metabolomics, and interventions to elucidate the metabolic interactions between the gut microbes and the host. Importantly, implementation of standardized approaches for fecal sample processing and microbiome assays is highly needed to enable reliable comparisons across different studies. In conclusion, there is now evidence that the gut microbiota associates with many of the complex metabolic abnormalities of obesity. It is, however, too early to conclude whether dysbiosis represents a causal factor in the pathogenesis of obesity and thus a new therapeutic target in prevention and treatment of obesity and its complications.

References

1. Diamant M, Blaak EE, de Vos WM. Do nutrient-gut-microbiota interactions play a role in human obesity, insulin resistance and type 2 diabetes? Obes Rev. 2011;12:272–81.
2. Backhed F, Ley RE, Sonnenburg JL, Peterson DA, Gordon JI. Host-bacterial mutualism in the human intestine. Science. 2005;307: 1915–20.
3. Gill SR, Pop M, Deboy RT, Eckburg PB, Turnbaugh PJ, Samuel BS, et al. Metagenomic analysis of the human distal gut microbiome. Science. 2006;312:1355–9.
4. Musso G, Gambino R, Cassader M. Interactions between gut microbiota and host metabolism predisposing to obesity and diabetes. Annu Rev Med. 2011;62:361–80.
5. Peterson J, Garges S, Giovanni M, McInnes P, Wang L, Schloss JA, et al. The NIH human microbiome project. Genome Res. 2009;19: 2317–23.
6. Spor A, Koren O, Ley R. Unravelling the effects of the environment and host genotype on the gut microbiome. Nat Rev Microbiol. 2011;9:279–90.

7. Qin J, Li R, Raes J, Arumugam M, Burgdorf KS, Manichanh C, et al. A human gut microbial gene catalogue established by metagenomic sequencing. Nature. 2010;464:59–65.

8. Claesson MJ, Jeffery IB, Conde S, Power SE, O'Connor EM, Cusack S, et al. Gut microbiota composition correlates with diet and health in the elderly. Nature. 2012;488:178–84.

9. Walker AW, Ince J, Duncan SH, Webster LM, Holtrop G, Ze X, et al. Dominant and diet-responsive groups of bacteria within the human colonic microbiota. ISME J. 2011;5:220–30.

10. Dethlefsen L, Huse S, Sogin ML, Relman DA. The pervasive effects of an antibiotic on the human gut microbiota, as revealed by deep 16S rRNA sequencing. PLoS Biol. 2008;6:e280.

11. Ley RE, Turnbaugh PJ, Klein S, Gordon JI. Microbial ecology: human gut microbes associated with obesity. Nature. 2006; 444:1022–3.

12. Turnbaugh PJ, Hamady M, Yatsunenko T, Cantarel BL, Duncan A, Ley RE, et al. A core gut microbiome in obese and lean twins. Nature. 2009;457:480–4.

13. Turnbaugh PJ, Ley RE, Mahowald MA, Magrini V, Mardis ER, Gordon JI. An obesity-associated gut microbiome with increased capacity for energy harvest. Nature. 2006;444: 1027–31.

14. Jumpertz R, Le DS, Turnbaugh PJ, Trinidad C, Bogardus C, Gordon JI, et al. Energy-balance studies reveal associations between gut microbes, caloric load, and nutrient absorption in humans. Am J Clin Nutr. 2011;94:58–65.

15. Erridge C, Attina T, Spickett CM, Webb DJ. A high-fat meal induces low-grade endotoxemia: evidence of a novel mechanism of postprandial inflammation. Am J Clin Nutr. 2007;86: 1286–92.

16. Backhed F, Manchester JK, Semenkovich CF, Gordon JI. Mechanisms underlying the resistance to diet-induced obesity in germ-free mice. Proc Natl Acad Sci U S A. 2007;104:979–84.

17. Cani PD, Possemiers S, Van de Wiele T, Guiot Y, Everard A, Rottier O, et al. Changes in gut microbiota control inflammation in obese mice through a mechanism involving GLP-2-driven improvement of gut permeability. Gut. 2009;58:1091–103.

18. Trasande L, Blustein J, Liu M, Corwin E, Cox LM, Blaser MJ. Infant antibiotic exposures and early-life body mass. Int J Obes (Lond). 2013;37:16–23.

19. Cho I, Yamanishi S, Cox L, Methe BA, Zavadil J, Li K, et al. Antibiotics in early life alter the murine colonic microbiome and adiposity. Nature. 2012;488:621–6.

20. Backhed F, Ding H, Wang T, Hooper LV, Koh GY, Nagy A, et al. The gut microbiota as an environmental factor that regulates fat storage. Proc Natl Acad Sci U S A. 2004;101:15718–23.

21. Vrieze A, Van Nood E, Holleman F, Salojarvi J, Kootte RS, Bartelsman JF, et al. Transfer of intestinal microbiota from lean donors increases insulin sensitivity in individuals with metabolic syndrome. Gastroenterology. 2012;143:913–16.
22. Delzenne NM, Neyrinck AM, Backhed F, Cani PD. Targeting gut microbiota in obesity: effects of prebiotics and probiotics. Nat Rev Endocrinol. 2011;7:639–46.

Chapter 11
Saturated Fat in Cardiovascular Disease and Obesity: Friend or Foe?

Aseem Malhotra

Saturated fat has been demonized ever since Ancel Keys' [1] landmark Seven Countries Study paper in 1970. It concluded that the incidence of coronary heart disease was directly related to serum cholesterol, which was directly related to the average proportions of calories provided by saturated fats in the diet of the cohorts in the study. It is important to note that this was not a robust dietary study and without making any allegations of causation suggested some associations. Nevertheless, it was the key paper in influencing a shift in dietary advice from "farinaceous and vegetable foods are fattening and saccharine matters are especially so" to "reduce fat intake to 30 % of total energy and a fall in saturated fat intake to 10 %" in the USA [2] and UK in 1977 and 1984, respectively [3]. Despite dietary advice influenced by the aforementioned findings, prospective cohort studies have not supported any significant association between saturated fat intake and risk of cardiovascular disease (CVD) [4]. Conversely Mozaffarian et al. [5] demonstrated dietary saturated fat to be inversely associated with coronary atherosclerosis progression in a cohort of postmenopausal women. More recently, a study by Otto et al. [6] looked into

A. Malhotra, MBCHR, MRCP (UK)
Department of Cardiology, Royal Free University Hospital,
Pond Street, Hampstead, London, NW3 2QG, UK
e-mail: aseem.malhotra@hotmail.com

D.W. Haslam et al. (eds.), *Controversies in Obesity*,
DOI 10.1007/978-1-4471-2834-2_11,
© Springer-Verlag London 2014

whether different food sources of saturated fat may influence the incidence of CVD events in a multiethnic population, revealing that a higher intake of dairy saturated fat was associated with lower CVD risk, but not from meat intake. It is important to note that red meat and dairy products are the two major sources of saturated fat in the USA. Micha R et al. [7] concluded that consumption of processed meats but not red meat was associated with CHD and diabetes mellitus. The authors suggest an explanation for this finding is the harmful effects of nitrates and sodium as preservatives in the former.

The effect of dietary saturated fat that has been thought to have the greatest influence on CVD risk is elevated LDL cholesterol concentrations [8]; however, the reduction in LDL cholesterol from reducing saturated fat intake appears to be more specific to larger, more buoyant particles [9] when in fact it is the smaller and more dense LDL particles that have been implicated in influencing atherosclerotic CVD [10]. There is universal consensus from researchers that trans fats are detrimental to health and may even have an adverse effect on markers of inflammation and increase CVD risk in the short term [11], but there is no consistent evidence that saturated fat from non-processed foods is detrimental to health and may even be beneficial. Dairy foods are exemplary providers of vitamins A and D of which the UK is deficient [12]. As well as vitamin D deficiency being linked to a significantly increased risk of cardiovascular mortality, calcium and phosphorus found commonly in dairy foods may have antihypertensive effects that may contribute to inverse associations with CVD risk [13–15]. The cardiovascular health study revealed that higher concentrations of plasma trans-palmitoleic acid, a fatty acid mainly found in dairy foods, have been recently associated with higher HDL, lower triglycerides, lower CRP, reduced insulin resistance, and lower incident of diabetes type 1 adults [16]. Thus, through decades of victimizing saturated fat, the consumption of carbohydrates and sugar has been inadvertently promoted often added as a substitute for fat in many processed foods marketed as "low fat" or "fat free."

The benefits of low-carbohydrate diets in respect to weight loss have been increasingly incorporated in dietary advice for this purpose such as the ever popular Atkins [17] diet. Such diets have also been shown to improve all the components of atherogenic dyslipidemia [18]. Robert Lustig [19] has recently highlighted the toxicity of sugar in driving the metabolic syndrome. He also describes a biochemical basis for sugar reducing satiety by interfering with the transport and signalling of the hormone leptin and reducing dopamine signalling in the brain's reward center, compelling the individual to consume more. In relation to weight gain, fat has received notoriety based on its higher calorie content per gram in comparison to protein and carbohydrate. However, work by biochemist Richard Feinman [20] and nuclear physicist Eugene Fine on thermodynamics and the metabolic advantage of different diet compositions demonstrated that the body does not metabolize different macronutrients in the same way. One of the earliest obesity experiments was carried out by Kekwick [21] and Pawan, published in the Lancet in 1956. They compared groups consuming diets of 90 % fat versus 90 % protein versus 90 % carbohydrate and revealed the greatest weight loss in the fat-consuming group. The authors concluded that the "composition of the diet appeared to outweigh in importance the intake of calories." Most recently, the calorie is not a calorie theory has been further substantiated by a recent study published in JAMA, which revealed a low-fat diet showed the greatest decrease in energy expenditure, an unhealthy lipid pattern, and increased insulin resistance in comparison to a low-carbohydrate diet [22].

There is increasing evidence suggesting the disassociation between the consumption of saturated fat and the cause of heart disease and obesity. Despite the research supporting this argument, there continues to be an overemphasis on reduced-fat diets by the medical establishment.

Editorial Comment

Until the end of the eighteenth century, diabetes was generally assumed to be a disease of the kidneys, assumed to be to blame because of the amount of sugar they either leaked or secreted into the urine, causing it to taste sweet. Thomas Willis, famous for describing the Circle of Willis, recognized the sweet taste of urine in the condition he named "pissing evil." He wrote, "the urine is wonderfully sweet, as if it were imbued with honey or sugar," but didn't realize that the urine actually contained sugar: "it seems more hard to demonstrate, why the Piss of such as are sick of this Distemper, is so wonderfully sweet, or should taste like Honey.... why it should be so wonderfully sweet, like Sugar or Honey, is a knot not easy to untie." In the last decades of the eighteenth century, debate raged among the great European medical men, as to the causes and best treatments for diabetes. The traditional approach was to replace the sugar lost in urine by prescribing a high-sugar diet, a notion which sounds impossibly ludicrous today.

The Swiss anatomist Johann Brunner discovered the effect of removing a dog's pancreas, noting that on the fourth day "he was thirsty & drank exceedingly from a brook flowing past the town." However, Brunner didn't associate the symptoms with diabetes. Later, Matthew Dobson presented the case of Peter Dickonson, admitted into his Infirmary in 1772, passing 28 pints of urine per day. Dobson made the observation that on evaporation of the urine, a granulated white cake, indistinguishable from sugar, remained. Furthermore, Dobson also detected sweetness on tasting his patient's serum, which was "sweetish, but I thought, not so sweet as the urine" – the discovery of hyperglycemia. He concluded that "this saccharine matter was not formed in the secretory organ [kidney], but previously existed in the serum of the blood." The Portuguese doctors Amatus Lusitanus and Abraham Zacutus believed that eating too much was the cause of diabetes, Zacutus even suggesting that the stomach was disordered, a view shared by Thomas Sydenham, but neither proved it. In 1797 diabetes was finally proved to be a disease, not of the kidneys, but of the gastrointestinal tract, by the Physician to the Artillery, Scottish physician John Rollo. Rollo studied one of his officers, a Captain Meredith, corpulent sufferer from diabetes, by boiling down his 24-h urine output to sugar and assessing the amount he discovered with the amount of refined carbohydrate starch in his diet, documenting the correlation between increased dietary "farinaceous" starch and increased glycosuria. Rollo successfully managed Meredith by restricting dietary carbohydrate, becoming the first proponent of low-carbohydrate, high-protein diets in diabetes and obesity. "The cure of the disease is accomplished by regimen and medicines preventing the formation of sugar... an entire abstinence from every species of vegetable matter or a diet solely of animal food." Clearly the diet needed some refinement, and the clinicians Claude Bernard, William Harvey, and the undertaker to the Royal Family William Banting may take credit for the many advances (Bantin's diet in particular recommended 8 units of alcohol per day).

The low-carbohydrate approach became standard management of diabetes and obesity, so much that any major endocrinology textbook up until the mid-1950s recommended their use as a matter of course. The accompanying article discusses the Seven Countries Study and how misclassification of foods such as cakes and biscuits as saturated fat, rather than carbohydrate, has led to recent guidelines, food pyramids, and in the UK, the Eatwell Plate, to promote dietary regimes vastly overloaded with carbohydrates, which is as ludicrous as feeding sugar to diabetic patients, as was done up to the eighteenth century.

Modern evidence, such as A TO Z and the DIRECT study, backs up what Rollo discovered in 1797, albeit by using more scientifically validated low-carbohydrate approaches; but it is likely that reliance on low-fat diets, in particular, as are still promoted widely, has caused unimaginable harm.

References

1. Keys A. Coronary heart disease in seven countries. Circulation. 1970;41(Supp):1–211.
2. Carter JP. Eating in America; Dietary Goals for the United States. Report of the Select Committee on Nutrition and Human Needs, U.S. Senate. Cambridge: MIT Press; 1977.
3. Diet and cardiovascular disease. Committee on Medical Aspects of Food Policy. Report of the Panel on Diet in Relation to Cardiovascular Disease. Rep Health Soc Subj (Lond). 1984;28:1–32.

4. Siri-Tarino PW, Sun Q, Hu FB, Krauss RM. Meta-analysis of prospective cohort studies evaluating the association of saturated fat with cardiovascular disease. Am J Clin Nutr. 2010;91:535–46.
5. Mozaffarian D, Rimm EB, Herrington DM. Dietary fats, carbohydrate, and progression of coronary atherosclerosis in post-menopausal women. Am J Clin Nutr. 2004;80:1175–84.
6. de Marcia C, Oliveira Otto MC, Mozaffarian D, Kromhout D, Bertoni AG, Sibley CT, et al. Dietary intake of saturated fat by food source and incident cardiovascular disease: the Multi-Ethnic Study of Atherosclerosis. Am J Clin Nutr. 2012;96(2):397–404.
7. Micha R, Wallace SK, Mozaffarian D. Red and processed meat consumption and risk of incident coronary heart disease, stroke and diabetes mellitus: a systematic review and meta analysis. Circulation. 2010;121:2271–83.
8. Dreon DM, Fernstrom HA, Campos H, Blanche P, Williams PT, Krauss RM. Change in dietary saturated fat intake is correlated with change in mass of large low-density-lipoprotein particles in men. Am J Clin Nutr. 1998;67:828–36.
9. Mensink RP, Katan MB. Effect of dietary fatty acids on serum lipids and lipoproteins: a meta-analysis of 27 trials. Arterioscler Thromb. 1992;12:911–9.
10. Berneis KK, Krauss RM. Metabolic origins and clinical significance of LDL heterogeneity. J Lipid Res. 2002;43:1363–79.
11. Wallace S, Mozaffarian D. Trans-fatty acids and non lipid risk factors. Curr Atheroscler Rep. 2009;11:423.
12. A UK National Statistics Publication. Family food. London: Department for Environment, Food and Rural Affairs; 2010.
13. Alonso A, Nettleton JA, Ix JH, de Boer IH, Folsom AR, Bidulescu A, et al. Dietary phosphorus, blood pressure and incidence of hypertension in the atherosclerosis risk in communities study and the multi-ethnic study of atherosclerosis. Hypertension. 2010;55:776–84.
14. Sacks FM, Willett WC, Smith A, Brown LE, Rosner B, Moore TJ. Effect on blood pressure of potassuim, calcium, and magnesium in women with low habitual intake. Hypertension. 1998;31:131–8.
15. Geleiijnse JM, Kok FJ, Grobee DE. Blood pressure response to changes in sodium and potassium intake: a metaregression analysis of randomised trials. J Hum Hypertens. 2003;17:471–80.
16. Mozaffarian D, Cao H, King IB, Lemaitre RN, Song X, Siscovick DS, et al. Trans. – Palmitoleic acid, metabolic risk factors, and new-onset diabetes in U.S adults: a cohort study. Ann Intern Med. 2010; 153:790–9.
17. Atkins RC. Dr. Atkins' new diet revolution. New York: Avon Books; 2002.
18. Krauss RM, Blanche PJ, Rawlings RS, Fernstrom HS, Williams PT. Separate effects of reduced carbohydrate intake and weight loss on atherogenic dyslipidemia. Am J Clin Nutr. 2006;83:1025–31; quiz 1205.

19. Lustig RH, Schmidt L, Brindis C. The toxic truth about sugar. Nature. 2012;482:27–9.
20. Feinman R, Fine E. A calorie is a calorie violates the second law of thermodynamics. Nutr J. 2004;3:9.
21. Kekwick A, Pawan GL. Calorie intake in relation to body-weight changes in the obese. Lancet. 1956;271(6935):155–61.
22. Ebbeling CB, Swain JF, Feldman HA, Wong WW, Hachey DL, Garcia-Lago E, et al. Effects of dietary composition on energy expenditure during weight-loss maintenance. JAMA. 2012;307(24): 2627–34.

Chapter 12
Childhood Obesity
and the Environment

Paul A. Whaley

Perhaps the biggest challenge to conventional explanations for the fattening of the population is the growing epidemic of obesity among infants [1]. Since infants have neither ever had much of an exercise regime nor eaten much other than breast milk or formula, the standard explanations for the rise in incidence of obesity, of sedentary lifestyle and poor diet, does not work for babies. Research into changes to the prenatal environment is therefore of particular interest.

Two obvious changes in the prenatal environment require acknowledgement. First is the trend towards maternal overweight, with predictions that 22 % of UK mothers by 2010 would have been obese at the start of pregnancy [2], a growing and recognized risk factor in infant overweight [3]. Second is increasing maternal age at pregnancy, which carries a higher risk of a range of complications [4], though specific research into the effect of maternal age at conception on infant weight gain seems to be limited.

A third factor that has more recently begun competing for attention as a contributor to the obesity epidemic is exposure to so-called chemical obesogens. While the possibility that chemicals may make people fatter has formed part of research recommendations in US First Lady Michelle

P.A. Whaley, BA, MLitt
Cancer Prevention and Education Society,
6 West Street, Axminster, Devon, EX13 5NX, UK
e-mail: pwhaley@cancerpreventionsociety.org

D.W. Haslam et al. (eds.), *Controversies in Obesity*,
DOI 10.1007/978-1-4471-2834-2_12,
© Springer-Verlag London 2014

Obama's campaign to reduce child obesity [5], others have described the hypothesis as a "green scare" and a subversion of "serious discussion" of how to reduce rates of obesity [6].

From a scientific perspective, it may be hasty to dismiss the obesogen hypothesis as a subversion or a scare. It is already recognized that the prenatal environment can modify obesity risk, from the discovery that children conceived during conditions of famine are more likely to suffer metabolic disorders later in life [7, 8]. It is also known that at least some prenatal chemical exposures can raise the risk of childhood obesity, as women who smoke while pregnant are more likely to have obese children [9], with nicotine identified as the likely causative agent [10].

Glucocorticoid, sex steroid, thyroid peroxisome proliferator-activated receptors (PPARs), and the retinoid X receptors (RXRs) all play prominent roles in regulating adipogenesis, lipid metabolism, metabolic set points, and adipose remodeling [11]; exogenous agents that interact with these receptors can reasonably be hypothesized to affect risk of obesity.

Proof of concept is again readily available: thiazolidinedione drugs, used for glycemic control in diabetes, are already recognized pharmaceutical obesogens, inducing weight gain via agonism of PPARγ [12]. Experimental data in animals suggest other mechanisms by which brief chemical exposure early in development can increase weight gain later on. For example, by the age of 6 months, mice treated at birth with the estrogenic drug diethylstilboestrol (DES) have considerably larger fat mass than untreated controls, with no evidence of changes in feeding habits or physical activity [13], suggesting that DES exposure sets a mouse's metabolism to conserve energy, predisposing it towards obesity in a food-rich environment.

The real controversy, of course, is whether or not ordinary human exposure to chemicals in the environment, from sources such as diet, consumer products, and air pollution, might contribute to an obesogenic prenatal environment.

Some of the most detailed research has been carried out on tributyltin (TBT), an organotin antifouling agent particularly toxic to molluscs, with just 2.4 ng/l of TBT sufficient to induce imposex in dog whelks [14]. TBT binds to the RXR-PPARγ heterodimer; when murine multipotent stromal stem cells (MSSCs), derived from 8-week-old animals exposed in utero to TBT or PPARγ agonists, are subjected to a subsequent in vitro challenge, they are twice as likely to become fat cells than bone cells [15]. Although TBT is rarely detected in human samples, when it is found its levels are in a range sufficient for effective receptor activation [12].

Bisphenol A, a ubiquitous environmental estrogen prominent in food packaging, interferes with the function of mouse pancreatic cells [16] and affects adipogenesis [17]. Epidemiological evidence is beginning to emerge associating BPA exposure with increased waist circumference in both Chinese [18] and US populations [19], though the direction of causation is unresolved. There is some evidence that phthalates [20] and stain-repellent perfluorinated compounds [21] may also be obesogenic.

Obesity is not only a health problem in and of itself; it is of concern to the medical and public health communities because of the health problems that come with it, with diabetes a particular health risk in obese people. As with obesity, exposure to chemicals in the environment complicates the standard account that diabetes rates are rising because an aging population, predisposed towards diabetes, is leading an increasingly sedentary lifestyle and eating more foods high in animal fats.

Human epidemiological studies are showing consistent correlations between type 2 diabetes and exposure to persistent organic pollutants (POPs) such as DDT, PCBs, and dioxins [22]. Early research found that levels of PCBs among subjects with diabetes were 30 % higher than in control subjects [23], while prospective epidemiological studies have reinforced the suggestion that POP exposure is a causal factor in the onset of type 2 diabetes [24, 25]. One particularly provocative study found that background levels of POPs are sufficient to induce diabetes in obese people [26]. If true, this would be a significant confounder in epidemiological identification of obesity as a factor in the etiology of diabetes, and it would have to be countenanced that obesity may only be a risk factor for diabetes in conjunction with POPs exposure [27].

Chemical exposures also threaten the simplicity of our understanding of the relationship between obesity and cancer. Not only is BPA a potential obesogen, as an environmental estrogen there are concerns it can modify risk of hormone-related cancers: BPA exposure in mice remodels' breast tissue in a manner associated with carcinogenesis in rodents and humans [28] and (again in a mouse model) seems to promote cancer cell growth and reduce the ability of breast tissue to defend against carcinogenic insults [29].

Research into obesogens is still very much in its early stages. Little is known about people's exposure to obesogens or which chemicals are problematic, partly because no chemical has ever been tested for obesogenicity before being brought to market. In the context of modern, calorie-dense diets and increasingly sedentary lifestyles, however, the possibility that some chemicals may be loading the dice against public health weight-loss initiatives makes the obesogen hypothesis look like an issue worth investigating.

References

1. Kim J, Peterson KE, Scanlon KS, Fitzmaurice GM, Must A, Oken E, et al. Trends in overweight from 1980 through 2001 among preschool-aged children enrolled in a health maintenance organization. Obesity (Silver Spring). 2006;14(7):1107–12.
2. Heslehurst N, Ells LJ, Simpson H, Batterham A, Wilkinson J, Summerbell CD. Trends in maternal obesity incidence rates, demographic predictors, and health inequalities in 36,821 women over a 15-year period. BJOG. 2007;114(2):187–94.
3. Dennedy MC, Avalos G, O'Reilly MW, O'Sullivan EP, Dunne FP. The impact of maternal obesity on gestational outcomes. Ir Med J. 2012;105(5 Suppl):23–5.
4. Johnson J, Tough S. Delayed child-bearing. J Obstet Gynaecol Can. 2012;34(1):80–93.
5. White House Task Force on Childhood Obesity. Solving the problem of childhood obesity within a generation. United States. 2010. http://www.letsmove.gov/sites/letsmove.gov/files/TaskForce_on_Childhood_Obesity_May2010_FullReport.pdf.
6. Finley A. Are plastics making us fat? Health gurus claim chemicals—not calories—are the cause of obesity. Wall Street Journal, United States 13/8/10. Cited 12/12/12. http://online.wsj.com/article/SB10001424052748703545604575407201305888876.html

7. de Rooij SR, Painter RC, Holleman F, Bossuyt PM, Roseboom TJ. The metabolic syndrome in adults prenatally exposed to the Dutch famine. Am J Clin Nutr. 2007;86(4):1219–24.

8. Li Y, Jaddoe VW, Qi L, He Y, Wang D, Lai J, et al. Exposure to the chinese famine in early life and the risk of metabolic syndrome in adulthood. Diabetes Care. 2011;34(4):1014–8.

9. Monasta L, Batty GD, Cattaneo A, Lutje V, Ronfani L, van Lenthe FJ, et al. Early-life determinants of overweight and obesity: a review of systematic reviews. Obes Rev. 2010;11(10):695–708.

10. Thayer KA, Heindel JJ, Bucher JR, Gallo MA. Role of environmental chemicals in diabetes and obesity: a National Toxicology Program workshop review. Environ Health Perspect. 2012;120(6):779–89.

11. Grün F, Blumberg B. Perturbed nuclear receptor signaling by environmental obesogens as emerging factors in the obesity crisis. Rev Endocr Metab Disord. 2007;8(2):161–71.

12. Grün F. Obesogens. Curr Opin Endocrinol Diabetes Obes. 2010;17(5):453–9.

13. Newbold RR, Padilla-Banks E, Jefferson WN. Environmental estrogens and obesity. Mol Cell Endocrinol. 2009;304(1–2):84–9.

14. International Maritime Organization. Anti-fouling systems. London; 2002.

15. Kirchner S, Kieu T, Chow C, Casey S, Blumberg B. Prenatal exposure to the environmental obesogen tributyltin predisposes multipotent stem cells to become adipocytes. Mol Endocrinol. 2010;24(3):526–39.

16. Alonso-Magdalena P, Morimoto S, Ripoll C, Fuentes E, Nadal A. The estrogenic effect of bisphenol A disrupts pancreatic beta-cell function in vivo and induces insulin resistance. Environ Health Perspect. 2006;114(1):106–12.

17. Somm E, Schwitzgebel VM, Toulotte A, Cederroth CR, Combescure C, Nef S, et al. Perinatal exposure to bisphenol a alters early adipogenesis in the rat. Environ Health Perspect. 2009;117(10):1549–55.

18. Wang H, Zhou Y, Tang C, Wu J, Chen Y, Jiang Q. Association between bisphenol a exposure and body mass index in Chinese school children: a cross-sectional study. Environ Health. 2012;11(1):79.

19. Trasande L, Attina TM, Blustein J. Association between urinary bisphenol A concentration and obesity prevalence in children and adolescents. JAMA. 2012;308(11):1113–21.

20. Stahlhut RW, van Wijngaarden E, Dye TD, Cook S, Swan SH. Concentrations of urinary phthalate metabolites are associated with increased waist circumference and insulin resistance in adult U.S. males. Environ Health Perspect. 2007;115(6):876–82.

21. Vanden Heuvel JP, Thompson JT, Frame SR, Gillies PJ. Differential activation of nuclear receptors by perfluorinated fatty acid analogs and natural fatty acids: a comparison of human, mouse, and rat

peroxisome proliferator-activated receptor-alpha, -beta, and -gamma, liver X receptor-beta, and retinoid X receptor-alpha. Toxicol Sci. 2006;92(2):476–89.

22. Carpenter DO. Environmental contaminants as risk factors for developing diabetes. Rev Environ Health. 2008;23(1):59–74.

23. Longnecker MP, Klebanoff MA, Brock JW, Zhou H. Polychlorinated biphenyl serum levels in pregnant subjects with diabetes. Diabetes Care. 2001;24(6):1099–101.

24. Turyk M, Anderson H, Knobeloch L, Imm P, Persky V. Organochlorine exposure and incidence of diabetes in a cohort of Great Lakes sport fish consumers. Environ Health Perspect. 2009;117(7):1076–82.

25. Rignell-Hydbom A, Lidfeldt J, Kiviranta H, Rantakokko P, Samsioe G, Agardh C, et al. Exposure to p, p′-DDE: a risk factor for type 2 diabetes. PLoS One. 2009;4(10):e7503.

26. Lee D, Steffes MW, Sjödin A, Jones RS, Needham LL, Jacobs DR. Low dose of some persistent organic pollutants predicts type 2 diabetes: a nested case–control study. Environ Health Perspect. 2010;118(9):1235–42.

27. Lee D, Jacobs DR, Porta M. Could low-level background exposure to persistent organic pollutants contribute to the social burden of type 2 diabetes? J Epidemiol Community Health. 2006;60(12):1006–8.

28. Markey CM, Luque EH, Munoz De Toro M, Sonnenschein C, Soto AM. In utero exposure to bisphenol A alters the development and tissue organization of the mouse mammary gland. Biol Reprod. 2001;65(4):1215–23.

29. Weber Lozada K, Keri RA. Bisphenol A increases mammary cancer risk in two distinct mouse models of breast cancer. Biol Reprod. 2011;85(3):490–7.

Chapter 13
Genetics and Epigenetics: Myths or Facts?

Kirsi H. Pietiläinen

It Is in My Genes

Overweight subjects often feel that the problem is that obesity runs in their family. By this they mean the genetic aggregation of obesity, not the equally likely possibility that no one runs in their family. Genetic influences of obesity were not generally accepted until Professor Albert J. Stunkard in the mid-1980s showed through large population-based twin and adoption studies that genetic factors do indeed play an important role in human obesity. The classical twin studies, comparing the similarity of monozygotic (MZ) and dizygotic (DZ) twins, estimated very high levels of heritability for body mass index (BMI), up to 80 % [1]. Because twins raised together may follow similar eating and exercise habits, a common criticism for twin studies is the possibility of equal environments rather than genes causing the phenotypic similarities. However, heritability of BMI in twins who have been reared apart is only slightly lower (70 %) [2] than in twins reared together, suggesting that these estimates are not biased upwards due to early shared environment. Anecdotal

K.H. Pietiläinen, MD, PhD, MSc in Nutrition
Obesity Research Unit, Biomedicum Helsinki,
University of Helsinki and Central Hospital,
Haartmaninkatu 8, Room C424,
700, Helsinki 00029, Finland
e-mail: kirsi.pietilainen@helsinki.fi

D.W. Haslam et al. (eds.), *Controversies in Obesity*,
DOI 10.1007/978-1-4471-2834-2_13,
© Springer-Verlag London 2014

stories of MZ twins separated at birth, being adopted to different families, and reunited in adulthood also show that despite different family environments, most MZ twins live astonishingly identical lives, develop the same preferences, and end up with almost exactly the same body weight.

Further proof of a genetic contribution to obesity was demonstrated in the seminal paper on adult Danish adoptees, where the weight class of the adoptees was strongly related to the BMI of their biological parents, while no relation was found to the adoptive parents [3]. However, heritabilities of obesity from adoption and family studies are generally lower and much more variable (20–80 %) than those from twin studies. Therefore, there is also room for the belief of environmental over genetic explanation to obesity.

Or Is It in My Jeans?

There is a popular proverb stating that the dramatic worldwide increase in obesity prevalence must be due to changes in the environment because our genes have not changed during the last decades. At the same time, evidence exists that genetic influences on adiposity have in fact increased during the last 50 years [4]. Data on nearly 270,000 Swedish full brothers, including MZ and DZ twin pairs, show that the heritability has increased from 75 to 79 % over the years, with a simultaneous considerable increase in the *variance* of genetic effects [4]. This would imply that modern lifestyle with minimal constraints on energy intake allows full expression of obesity risk genes and that it is primarily the genetic background that creates the considerable variation in body fatness within populations living in obesogenic environments.

On the other hand, several recent studies have revealed that choosing a physically active lifestyle can counteract genetic obesity risk. In young adult Finnish twins, it was shown that while the heritability of BMI is over 80 % in the sedentary group, it was only about 60 % in the physically active group [5]. In line with this, studies using markers identified in genome-wide association studies (GWAS) have shown that physical activity attenuates the genetic predisposition to obesity by as much as 30–40 % [6, 7]. This suggests that it is possible to decrease the genetic susceptibility to obesity by increasing physical activity.

Good Appetite or Poor Metabolism?

Having a lazy metabolism, naturally for genetic reasons, is an attractive explanation for obesity. However, genetic studies, neither in the candidate gene nor in the GWAS era, do not support this hypothesis. Frankly, this phenotype has not been extensively studied because, until now, large enough data for molecular genetic studies have not existed. Most genes – to date, over 50 – unequivocally associating to adiposity seem to regulate eating and appetite [8]. This is especially the case for the two major contributors of polygenic variation in obesity, *FTO* and *MC4R*.

Missing Heritability

Despite the accelerated gene discovery, the established loci are able to explain only a fraction (5 %) of the heritability of obesity [8]. Where is all the rest of the heritability? Twin studies suggest that if you would have a complete copy of yourself with all the 20,000 genes, all their interactions with each other and with the prevailing environment, the two of you would almost certainly have similar body weights. It may then be that it is this network of interactions rather than individual genes that makes body weight so heritable and the billions of dynamic communications between molecules, cells, and organs that make understanding of the system so challenging. The lost heritability can also be found in the epigenetic mechanisms, such as DNA methylation or histone modification, which control how genes are activated in each circumstance.

Since epigenetic mechanisms themselves are controlled by genes, these intertwined processes together produce the highly transmissible phenotype.

Over and Above the Genes

If genetics is the writing "madamimadam," epigenetics provides the instructions on how to read it: "Madam, I'm Adam." Epigenetic errors can also change the readout: "Mad $_{amim}$ Adam," completely altering the function of the gene. Unlike the fixed DNA sequence in each of the over 200 different human cell types, epigenetic patterns may vary from tissue to tissue and are sensitive to environmental exposures. It is this propensity for change, promise of modifiable effects that has made the hype around epigenetic processes, the epidemic of epigenetics, the surge of review after review with very few actual data about the whole genome-scale epigenetic patterns in obesity.

Dolly, the Sheep, and Other Clonal Controls

As the cloning of Dolly in 1997 showed, we are more than our genes. Dolly was obese and had at least two obesity-related complications, arthritis and diabetes, unlike its genetically identical mother. Development of obesity in Dolly was clearly an epigenetic phenomenon. Genetically identical humans, MZ twins, discordant for body weight are very rare but ideal in the search for epigenetic alterations in obesity that are due to lifestyle or that are linked to the development of metabolic complications independent of genetic background. At the dawn of such studies, it is fair to assume that epigenetics can be used to identify early metabolic abnormalities because healthy and unhealthy obesity seem to create different epigenetic signatures (Ollikainen M et al., unpublished observations). Because the results point to nutritional pathways, it seems likely that the epigenetic modifications can be reversed by dietary approaches. Especially intriguing is the possibility that through epigenetic biomarkers, we can both find new diagnostics tools as well as targets to erase bad metabolic memories. If it is possible to nurture the nature of the peripheral tissues, is it possible to rewire the brain epigenetically to resist the temptations of the obesogenic environment?

Conclusion

Obesity is a result of genetic, epigenetic, and environmental factors, with numerous possible perturbations in the complex pathways leading to phenotypically very heterogeneous traits. Despite decades of intensive study, a fine-grained understanding of the mechanisms underlying regulation of body weight remains rather rudimentary. Future studies seeking to integrate networks of dynamic, functional data, including epigenetics, will be crucial in understanding the ultimate disease outcomes and their possible treatment. Be it fast food, slow motion, or lazy metabolism, molecular understanding of their mechanisms will teach us how human nature controls nurture and vice versa.

References

1. Stunkard AJ, Foch TT, Hrubec Z. A twin study of human obesity. JAMA. 1986;256:51–4.
2. Allison DB, Kaprio J, Korkeila M, Koskenvuo M, Neale MC, Hayakawa K. The heritability of body mass index among an international sample of monozygotic twins reared apart. Int J Obes Relat Metab Disord. 1996;20(6):501–6.
3. Stunkard AJ, Sørensen TIA, Hanis C, Teasdale TW, Chakraborty R, Schull WJ, et al. An adoption study of human obesity. N Engl J Med. 1986;314:193–8.
4. Rokholm B, Silventoinen K, Tynelius P, Gamborg M, Sørensen TI, Rasmussen F. Increasing genetic variance of body mass index during the Swedish obesity epidemic. PLoS One. 2011;6(11): e27135.

5. Mustelin L, Silventoinen K, Pietiläinen KH, Rissanen A, Kaprio J. Physical activity reduces the influence of genetic effects on BMI and waist circumference: a study in young adult twins. Int J Obes. 2009;33:29–36.

6. Li S, Zhao JH, Luan J, Ekelund U, Luben RN, Khaw KT, et al. Physical activity attenuates the genetic predisposition to obesity in 20,000 men and women from EPIC-Norfolk prospective population study. PLoS Med. 2010;7:pii: e1000332.

7. Kilpeläinen TO, Qi L, Brage S, Sharp SJ, Sonestedt E, Demerath E, et al. Physical activity attenuates the influence of FTO variants on obesity risk: a meta-analysis of 218,166 adults and 19,268 children. PLoS Med. 2011;8:e1001116.

8. Loos RJ. Genetic determinants of obesity and their value in prediction. Best Pract Res Clin Endocrinol Metab. 2012;26:211–22.

Chapter 14
Chronicities of Modernity and the Contained Body as an Explanation for the Global Pandemic of Obesity, Diabetes, and the Metabolic Syndrome

Dennis Wiedman

Introduction

With the diffusion of modernity throughout the world, we see the rise of the global pandemic of obesity, diabetes, and the metabolic syndrome. Throughout human evolution obesity was rare because seasonal variation in physical activities, and the foods we ate, promoted good cardiovascular and metabolic fitness. In more recent times, the kinds of work, foods consumed, cultural beliefs, and living and work spaces all pattern and routinize the modern body. Chronicities of Modernity Theory focuses on the sociocultural factors that structure an individual's everyday life, containing the physical body in

D. Wiedman, PhD Anthropology
Department of Global and Sociocultural Studies,
School of International and Public Affairs, SIPA 327,
Florida International University, 11200 SW 8th Street,
Miami, FL 33199, USA
e-mail: wiedmand@fiu.edu

D.W. Haslam et al. (eds.), *Controversies in Obesity*,
DOI 10.1007/978-1-4471-2834-2_14,
© Springer-Verlag London 2014

ways that increase the three risk factors for obesity, diabetes, and metabolic syndrome: (1) physical inactivity, (2) overnutrition, and (3) chronic stress. Each of these three risk factors alone does not fully explain metabolic syndrome; it is the conjuncture of these for a long duration in a person's life that are most predictive. Recurrent cognitive, social, and material processes of modernity become embodied into the physiology and metabolism of an individual's body during gestation, through early childhood, into adult and later years resulting in obesity and metabolic syndrome [1].

Beginning in the 1940s, American Indians and indigenous people in the South Pacific were first identified with this epidemic. By the late 1960s researchers began reporting that diabetes increased significantly as populations moved from rural to urban locations, migrated to developed nations, lived on the more acculturated Pacific islands, or American Indian reservations [2–6]. In 1971, diabetes was called the "Price of Civilization" [7]. Once a disease of indigenous peoples, ethnic minorities, and inner-city poor, obesity and metabolic syndrome now affect the full spectrum of social classes and ethnic groups in the developed and developing nations, with China, India, and the Middle East now experiencing the greatest increases [8, 9].

During the 1980s, obesity, diabetes, dyslipidemia, and hypertension were recognized as having similar metabolic defects [10, 11]. In 1999, the World Health Organization formulated a definition for the cluster of these disorders as the metabolic syndrome. In order to maintain proper body weight, currently the International Diabetes Federation recommends individuals to avoid eating foods high in sugars and saturated fats and to experience at least 30 min of moderate physical activity each day such as brisk walking, swimming, cycling, or dancing [12]. This is a shift in explanation from an emphasis on genetics and biomedical interventions to social and cultural factors that affect nutrition and physical activity.

Throughout human evolution, daily physical activity and periods of rest varied throughout the year in response to the demands of the food production cycle. Anthropomorphic data for the hunting and gathering Hadza of Tanzania [13] and agriculturalists of Benin [14] indicate that body mass index and percent body fat fluctuate seasonally with the amount of energy expended and available food resources. Ethnographic and archeological data indicate that most hunters and gatherers are physically active mobile populations using a wide variety of food resources, enabling them to exploit resources that are seasonally abundant in some areas while not abundant in others [15]. The feast and famine assumption of James Neel's "thrifty gene" hypothesis, where genes were selected for quickly metabolizing food into fat, is not supported by a meta-analysis of hunters, gatherers, and agriculturalists research [16–19]. During human evolution as hunters and gatherers, seasonal variation in physical activities, foods, and body weights was normal; chronic physical inactivity, overnutrition, and consistent annual body weight of modernity are actually abnormal. Chronicities of Modernity Theory stresses a social and cultural explanation rather than a genetic predisposition for these metabolic disorders. At the critical juncture with modernity, populations shift from seasonally variable physical activities and food resources to chronically low levels of physical activities, consistent caloric intake, and, for many groups, recurrent psychosocial stresses. In a study of 30 rural populations in developing countries, seasonal weight loss was the norm [20]. Alaska Natives living a hunting and fishing food production lifestyle that changes with the seasons have better physical and mental outcomes then their urban relatives [21–23]. Prolonged physical inactivity and rest of modernity produce the biochemical responses of metabolic syndrome [24]. Human and other mammal populations experience similar metabolic disorders with the shift from seasonality to chronicities of modernity. Cats confined indoors and captive marmosets in zoos also develop obesity and diabetes [25, 26]. These studies indicate that an annual variation in daily activities and foods is the normal human condition. Chronically low levels of physical activity and consistent sources of calories throughout the year are the abnormal human condition.

Socially constructed beliefs, practices, and material cultures of modernity contain the human body. These constraints and incentives set parameters and pattern an individual's decisions and behaviors. These "structural chronicities" do not affect all members of a society equally, but specific population segments, and these from country to country. Females often have higher prevalence rates, but in some nations it is the males. Once considered an adult disorder, it is now affecting children. Where inner-city uneducated poor were at highest risk, the well educated with higher incomes are now at risk. Urbanized areas have higher rates, but so do many rural areas and especially among Indigenous peoples on reservations. In order to better understand this variation from nation to nation, "structural chronicities" provide a cross-cultural way of identifying the most important structural factors and forces. For example, American Indian reservations imposed severe physical constraints on the Indigenous body; they were the earliest socially created built environments where generations of humans lived almost entirely on industrially processed energy-dense foods and where the entire population was held in chronic levels of stress [27]. In contrast to the economically poor conditions of Indian reservations, 25 % of the exceedingly wealthy Indigenous peoples of the United Arab Emirates are diagnosed with diabetes. Fifty years ago, as pastoralists annually migrating from the interior to the shore, they now live along the coast in modern homes and high-rise condominiums with few pedestrian walkways. Shopping malls are the most used public spaces for walking. To go somewhere they call a driver. They hire workers from other countries to do the physical labor, housework, and cooking. The sweet palm dates they once cultivated have culturally transformed into elaborate high-calorie chocolate gifts. Commensality and overeating food are central to their frequent family and social gatherings. Combined with these structures, stress from gender role expectations elevates the number of women with diabetes [28]. These two cases illustrate that income, education, power, and social class explanations do not sufficiently explain the causes of obesity and diabetes among populations of the world.

Structural chronicities of modernity restrict the decisions and alternatives that individuals can take to improve their physical and mental well-being. Chronicities of Modernity Theory refocuses the emphasis of health interventions primarily from individual education, counseling, and medication regimens to community, national, and global factors and forces. This is a shift from the individual to the structures over which they have very little control. There is a need to create ideologies, social institutions, nutritional sources, and built environments that facilitate rather than hinder variation in physical activity, foods, and body weights. "Chronicities of modernity," "structural chronicities," and the "contained body" provide a biocultural paradigm for linking macro sociocultural factors to individual life experiences and biological disorders. Using Chronicities of Modernity Theory, we can better conceptualize and identify the sociocultural chronicities that most contain specific populations and life situations causing obesity, diabetes, and the metabolic syndrome.

References

1. Wiedman D. Globalizing the chronicities of modernity: diabetes and the metabolic syndrome. In: Manderson L, Smith-Morris C, editors. Chronic conditions, fluid states: chronicity and the anthropology of illness. New Brunswick: Rutgers University Press; 2010. p. 18–53.
2. Cleave TL, Campbell GD. Diabetes, coronary thrombosis and saccharine disease. Bristol: John Wright and Sons; 1969.
3. Cohen AM, Teitelbaum A, Saliternik R. Genetics and diet as factors in development of diabetes mellitus. Metabolism. 1972;21:235–40.
4. Wise P, Edwards F, Thomas D. Hyperglycaemia in the urbanized aboriginal. Med J Aust. 1970;2:1001–6.
5. Wiedman D. Oklahoma Cherokee technological development and diabetes mellitus. In: Baer H, editor. Encounters with biomedicine: case studies in medical anthropology. New York: Gordon and Breech Science Publishing Company; 1987. p. 43–71.
6. Wiedman D. Adiposity or longevity: which factor accounts for the increase of type II diabetes mellitus when populations acculturate to an industrial technology? Med Anthropol. 1989;11(3):237–52.
7. Prior I. The price of civilization. Nutr Today. 1971;6:2–11.

8. Wang Y, Mi J, Shan X, Wang O, Ge K. Is China facing an obesity epidemic and the consequences? The trends in obesity and chronic disease. Int J Obes (Lond). 2007;31:177–88.

9. Hossain P, Kawar B, El Nahas M. Obesity and diabetes in the developing world – a growing challenge. N Engl J Med. 2007;356(3):213–5.

10. Reaven E. Role of insulin resistance in human disease. Diabetes. 1988;37:1595–607.

11. Weiss KM, Ferrell RE, Hanis CL. New world syndrome of metabolic diseases with a genetic and evolutionary basis. Yearbook of Phys Anthropol. 1984;27:153–78.

12. Management of diabetes. Brussels: International Diabetes Federation. Accessed 23 Sept 2012.

13. Marlowe F, Berbesque J. Tubers as fallback foods and their impact on hadza hunter-gatherers. Am J Phys Anthropol. 2009;140:751–8.

14. Schultink WJ, Klaver W, Van Wijk H, Van Raaij J, Hautvaast J. Body weight changes and basal metabolic rates of rural Beninese women during seasons with different energy intakes. Eur J Clin Nutr. 1990;44 Suppl 1:31–40.

15. Lee R. What hunters do for a living, or, how to make out on scarce resources. In: Lee R, Devore I, editors. Man the hunter. Chicago: Aldine Publishing Co; 1968. p. 30–48.

16. Neel JV. Diabetes mellitus: a "thrifty" genotype rendered detrimental by "progress". Am J Hum Genet. 1962;14:353–62.

17. Neel JV. The thrifty gene revisited. In: Kobberling J, Tattersall J, editors. The genetics of diabetes mellitus. New York: Academic; 1982.

18. Neel JV. The thrifty genotype in 1999. Nutr Rev. 1999;57:2–9.

19. Benyshek DC, Watson JT. Exploring the thrifty genotype's food-shortage assumptions: a cross cultural comparison of ethnographic accounts of food security among foraging and agricultural societies. Am J Phys Anthropol. 2006;131:120–6.

20. Ferro-Luzzi A, Branca F. Nutritional seasonality: the dimensions of the problem. In: Ulijaszek S, Strickland S, editors. Seasonality and human ecology. Cambridge, UK: Cambridge University Press; 1993. p. 149–65.

21. Smith J, Johnson P, Easton P, Wiedman D, Widmark EG. Food customs of Alaska women of childbearing age: the Alaska WIC healthy moms survey. Ecol Food Nutr. 2008;47:1–33.

22. Smith J, Saylor BL, Easton PS, Wiedman D. Measurable benefits of traditional food customs in the lives of rural and urban Alaska Inupiaq elders. Alaska J Anthropol. 2009;7(1):89–99.

23. Smith J, Easton PS, Saylor BL. Inupiaq elders study: aspects of aging among male and female elders. Int J Circumpolar Health. 2009;68(2):182–96.

24. Chakravarthy M, Booth F. Eating, exercise, and "thrifty" genotypes: connecting the dots toward an evolutionary understanding of modern chronic diseases. J Appl Physiol. 2004;96(1):3–10.

25. Rand J, Fleeman L, Farrow H, Appleton D, Lederer R. Canine and feline diabetes mellitus: nature or nurture. J Nutr. 2004;34:2072S–80S.
26. Power ML. The human obesity epidemic, the mismatch paradigm, and Our modern "captive" environment. Am J Human Biol. 2012;24(2):116–22.
27. Wiedman D. Native American embodiment of the chronicities of modernity: reservation food, diabetes and the metabolic syndrome among the Kiowa, Comanche and Apache. Med Anthropol Q. 2012;26(4):595–612.
28. Baglar R. "Oh God, save us from sugar": an ethnographic exploration of diabetes mellitus in the United Arab Emirates. Med Anthropol. 2013;32(2):109–25.

Part IV
Clinical

Chapter 15
Screening for Type 2 Diabetes

Laura J. Gray, Melanie J. Davies, and Kamlesh Khunti

Introduction

Type 2 diabetes mellitus (T2DM) is an important health problem and is associated with increased risk of cardiovascular disease [1, 2]. It is estimated that there are 183 million cases of undiagnosed diabetes worldwide [3]. T2DM is often asymptomatic, remaining undiagnosed and, therefore, untreated, with the onset occurring 4–7 years before diagnosis [4]. Randomized controlled trials have shown that T2DM can be prevented through lifestyle or pharmacological intervention

L.J. Gray, PhD (✉)
Department of Health Sciences,
University of Leicester,
Gwendolen Road, Leicester, Leicestershire LE5 4PW, UK
e-mail: lg48@le.ac.uk

M.J. Davies, MB, ChB, MD
K. Khunti, FRCGP, FRCP, MD, PhD
Diabetes Research Centre,
University of Leicester,
Leicester Diabetes Centre,
Leicester General Hospital,
Gwendolen Road, Leicester LE5 4PW, UK
e-mail: melanie.davies@uhl-tr.nhs.uk; e-mail: kk22@le.ac.uk

D.W. Haslam et al. (eds.), *Controversies in Obesity*,
DOI 10.1007/978-1-4471-2834-2_15,
© Springer-Verlag London 2014

in those at high risk [5]. Although there is some evidence that population-based primary prevention is both clinically and cost-effective [6, 7], these interventions have not been fully implemented in the real world and screening remains a controversial issue [8, 9]. Here we discuss some of the issues surrounding screening for T2DM.

Types of Screening

Screening can take a number of modalities; population-based offers screening to all those in a particular group, whereas targeted screening would focus on those at high risk of the condition. Opportunistic screening occurs at a time when people are seen, by health care professionals, for a reason other than the disorder in question. The ADDITION-Europe study used a number of screening methods for case detection of T2DM [10, 11]. The lowest uptake to screening was seen in the center using a population-based approach; 20.2 % of those invited attended [12]. Uptake was increased when a population was prescreened using a validated risk score – 73.5 %. Utilizing opportunistic screening also saw higher uptake rates – 80.7–95.1 %. The level of case detection was also increased through preselecting a higher risk group [11]. Two diabetes prevention trials carried out in the UK, in contrast, found that prescreening using a risk score did not increase uptake to the screening program but did increase the level of case detection [13]. These studies, however, used a very low level means of risk communication and were conducted in a multiethnic population that could have affected uptake. Further research into how to engage the public in a screening program is warranted.

Identification of Those at Risk

Recently, the National Institute for Health and Clinical Excellence (NICE) in the UK has recommended the use of risk scores prior to blood testing for identifying those at high risk [14]. A plethora of risk scores have been developed and validated over the past 10 years [15–17]. For example, the Leicester Risk Assessment and the FINDRISC score were designed as questionnaires to be completed without intervention from a heath care professional or medical tests [18, 19]. Scores that have been developed using cross-sectional data can predict prevalent undiagnosed disease (e.g., the Leicester and Cambridge risk scores [20, 21]) in contrast to scores that have been developed using longitudinal data, where incidence can be predicted (e.g., FINDRISC and the QDScore [22, 23]). The scores developed to date tend to be for a specific population as studies have found that scores that have been developed elsewhere and used on a different population tend to have low validity [24, 25]. The PREDICT 2 study is currently trying to develop a globally applicable screening model [26].

Multiphasic screening occurs when multiple conditions are assessed within a single program. An example of this is the NHS Health Checks Programme within the UK. Here all those aged 40–75 are invited every 5 years to assess their risk of cardiovascular disease and diabetes and given advice on how to reduce risk [27].

Blood Testing

Once someone has been identified at high risk, they then need to either receive a diagnostic test; in the case of T2DM, this would be either oral glucose tolerance tests (OGTT) or HbA1c. Recently the WHO recommended that the diagnostic criteria for T2DM be revised to include those with an HbA1c of ≥6.5 % [28, 29]. WHO found insufficient evidence to classify those at high risk of T2DM using HbA1c [29]; however, an international expert panel and ADA have suggested that ranges of 6.0–6.4 % and 5.7–6.0 % can be considered [30]. Based on the ADA criteria, up to two-thirds of the population could fall into this category, which would overwhelm prevention initiatives. However, moving away from the OGTT has the potential to increase uptake to screening and has been recommended by NICE. The OGTT is costly, time-consuming, and inconvenient [31] and a barrier to attending screening [32].

Cost-Effectiveness of Screening

Any screening program not only needs to assess the sensitivity and specificity of the program in terms of disease detection, but also the cost-effectiveness. Screening for those at risk of T2DM allows preventative interventions to be initiated that are known to be cost-effective in reducing progression rates to T2DM [5,33,34]. To date there have been no trials comparing screening to no screening in terms of T2DM. Therefore, the assessments of efficacy and cost-effectiveness are based primarily on modelling studies. One recent economic decision analysis model estimated that compared with no screening, the cost of screening for diabetes and impaired glucose tolerance followed by lifestyle interventions was £6,242 (€7,750; $9,750) for each quality-adjusted life year (QALY) gained [33]. A simulated study using the Archimedes model suggested that compared with no screening, screening for T2DM is cost-effective when started between the ages of 30 years and 45 years, with screening repeated every 3–5 years [35]. Another study assessed the cost per case detected for a range of screening scenarios. This study found that the least expensive strategies were those involving a practice-based risk score followed by a single blood test and finally a confirmatory OGTT [36].

Treatments

A prerequisite for any screening program is that there should be an effective treatment or intervention for patients identified through early detection. The ADDITION trial was a pragmatic cluster randomized trial in which 343 general practices were randomly assigned to screening of registered patients aged 40–69 years without known diabetes followed by routine care of diabetes or to screening followed by intensive treatment of multiple risk factors. The primary outcome was first cardiovascular event within 5 years. Although the trial showed small but significant benefits in terms of cardiovascular risk factors, there was no difference between the two groups in terms of cardiovascular event rates at 5 years [10]. This was the first trial to assess hard outcomes in a screen-detected group. A sub-study of the ADDITION trial carried out in Cambridge, UK, has 10-year follow-up data on the participants enrolled at this center; additionally, they have reported no difference in 10-year all-cause, cardiovascular- or diabetes-related mortality rates between those treated aggressively and those receiving standard care [37]. Previous modelling studies showed more positive results [38, 39].

Conclusion

Population-based screening for T2DM is currently not recommended and is a controversial issue. Studies have shown that screening can result in T2DM being identified on average 3.3 years earlier [40]. Earlier diagnosis and treatment do not seem to improve longer-term outcomes [10]. Screening for those at risk of T2DM should be recommended as it is well known that progression to T2DM can be prevented or at least delayed in this group [5]. Identification can be achieved in a cost-effective manner using risk scores [36]. Screening for T2DM may only be feasible as part of multiphasic approach such as the NHS Health Checks Programme.

In conclusion, screening for those at risk of T2DM is both cost-effective and effective in terms of delaying and preventing T2DM. To date, screening for T2DM alone has not been shown to be beneficial.

Acknowledgments KK (Chair) and MJD were members of the National Institute for Health and Clinical Excellence Guidance PH38: Preventing type 2 diabetes: risk identification and interventions for individuals at high risk. LJG, KK, and MJD are supported by the National Institute for Health Research Collaboration for Leadership in

Applied Health Research and Care (NIHR CLAHRC)-Leicestershire, Northamptonshire, and Rutland and The NIHR Leicester-Loughborough Diet, Lifestyle and Physical Activity Biomedical Research Unit, which is a partnership between University Hospitals of Leicester NHS Trust, Loughborough University, and the University of Leicester.

References

1. Levitan EB, Song Y, Ford ES, Liu S. Is nondiabetic hyperglycemia a risk factor for cardiovascular disease?: a meta-analysis of prospective studies. Arch Intern Med. 2004;164(19):2147–55.
2. Cortez-Dias N, Martins S, Belo A, Fiuza M, VALSIM. Prevalence, management and control of diabetes mellitus and associated risk factors in primary health care in Portugal. Rev Port Cardiol. 2010;29(4): 509–37.
3. Whiting DR, Guariguata L, Weil C, Shaw J. IDF diabetes atlas: global estimates of the prevalence of diabetes for 2011 and 2030. Diabetes Res Clin Pract. 2011;94(3):311–21.
4. Harris MI, Klein R, Welborn TA, Knuiman MW. Onset of NIDDM occurs at least 4–7 yr before clinical diagnosis. Diabetes Care. 1992;15(7): 815–9.
5. Gillies CL, Abrams KR, Lambert PC, Cooper NJ, Sutton AJ, Hsu RT, et al. Pharmacological and lifestyle interventions to prevent or delay type 2 diabetes in people with impaired glucose tolerance: systematic review and meta-analysis. BMJ. 2007;334(7588):299.
6. Knowler WC, Narayan KM, Hanson RL, Nelson RG, Bennett PH, Tuomilehto J. Preventing non-insulin-dependent diabetes. Diabetes. 1995;44:483–8.
7. Segal L, Dalton AC, Richardson J. Cost-effectiveness of the primary prevention of non-insulin dependent diabetes mellitus. Health Promot Int. 1998;13:197–209.
8. Khunti K, Davies MJ. Should we screen for type 2 diabetes? Yes. BMJ. 2012;345:e4514.
9. Goyder E, Irwig L, Payne N. Should we screen for type 2 diabetes? No. BMJ. 2012;345:e4516.
10. Griffin SJ, Borch-Johnsen K, Davies MJ, Khunti K, Rutten GE, Sandbæk A, et al. Effect of early intensive multifactorial therapy on 5-year cardiovascular outcomes in individuals with type 2 diabetes detected by screening (ADDITION-Europe): a cluster-randomised trial. Lancet. 2011;378(9786):156–67.
11. van den Donk M, Sandbaek A, Borch-Johnsen K, Lauritzen T, Simmons RK, Wareham NJ, et al. Screening for type 2 diabetes. Lessons from the ADDITION-Europe study. Diabet Med. 2011;28(11): 1416–24.

12. Webb DR, Gray LJ, Khunti K, Srinivasan B, Taub N, Campbell S, et al. Screening for diabetes using an oral glucose tolerance test within a western multi-ethnic population identifies modifiable cardiovascular risk: the ADDITION-Leicester study. Diabetologia. 2011;54(9):2237–46.

13. Gray LJ, Khunti K, Edwardson C, Goldby S, Henson J, Morris DH, et al. Implementation of the automated Leicester practice risk score in two diabetes prevention trials provides a high yield of people with abnormal glucose tolerance. Diabetologia. 2012;55(12): 3238–44.

14. Chatterton H, Younger T, Fischer A, Khunti K, Programme Development Group. Risk identification and interventions to prevent type 2 diabetes in adults at high risk: summary of NICE guidance. BMJ. 2012;12(345):e4624.

15. Collins GS, Mallett S, Omar O, Yu L. Developing risk prediction models for type 2 diabetes: a systematic review of methodology and reporting. BMC Med. 2011;9:103.

16. Buijsse B, Simmons RK, Griffin SJ, Schulze MB. Risk assessment tools for identifying individuals at risk of developing type 2 diabetes. Epidemiol Rev. 2011;33(1):46–62.

17. Noble D, Mathur R, Dent T, Meads C, Greenhalgh T. Risk models and scores for type 2 diabetes: systematic review. BMJ. 2011;343:d7163.

18. Gray LJ, Taub N, Khunti K, Gardiner E, Hiles S, Webb DR, et al. The Leicester risk assessment score for detecting undiagnosed type 2 diabetes and impaired glucose regulation for use in a multiethnic UK setting. Diabet Med. 2010;27(8):887–95.

19. Lindström J, Tuomilehto J. The diabetes risk score. Diabetes Care. 2003;26(3):725–31.

20. Gray LJ, Davies MJ, Hiles S, Taub N, Webb DR, Srinivasan BT, Khunti K. Detection of Impaired Glucose Regulation and/or Type 2 Diabetes Mellitus, using primary care electronic data, in a multiethnic UK community setting. Diabetologia. 2012;55(4):959–66.

21. Griffin SJ, Little PS, Hales CN, Kinmonth AL, Wareham NJ. Diabetes risk score: towards earlier detection of Type 2 diabetes in general practice. Diabetes Metab Res Rev. 2000;16(3):164–71.

22. Hippisley-Cox J, Coupland C, Robson J, Sheikh A, Brindle P. Predicting risk of type 2 diabetes in England and Wales: prospective derivation and validation of QDScore. Br Med J. 2009;388:b880.

23. Lindstrom J, Tuomilehto J. The diabetes risk score: a practical tool to predict type 2 diabetes risk. Diabetes Care. 2003;26(3):725–31.

24. Rathmann W, Martin S, Haastert B, Icks A, Holle R, Lowel H, et al. Performance of screening questionnaires and risk scores for undiagnosed diabetes: the KORA survey 2000. Arch Intern Med. 2005;165(4): 436–41.

25. Witte DR, Shipley MJ, Marmot MG, Brunner EJ. Performance of existing risk scores in screening for undiagnosed diabetes: an external validation study. Diabet Med. 2010;27(1):46.

26. Vistisen D, Lee CM, Colagiuri S, Borch-Johnsen K, Glümer C. A globally applicable screening model for detecting individuals with undiagnosed diabetes. Diabetes Res Clin Pract. 2012;95(3):432–8.

27. Walker N, Gardiner E, Davies M, Khunti K. The vascular risk assessment programme: implications for the delivery in primary care. Diabet Prim Care. 2009;11(4):209–15.

28. World Health Organisation. Definition, diagnosis, and classification of diabetes mellitus and its complications. Report of a WHO consultation. Part 1: diagnosis and classification of diabetes mellitus. Geneva: World Health Organisation; 1999.

29. World Health Organisation. Use of glycated haemoglobin (HbA1c) in the diagnosis of diabetes mellitus. Geneva: World Health Organisation; 2011.

30. American Diabetes Association Position statement. Standards of medical care in diabetes—2010. Diabetes Care. 2010;33 Suppl 1:S11–61.

31. Waugh N, Scotland G, McNamee P, Gillett M, Brennan A, Goyder E, et al. Screening for type 2 diabetes: literature review and economic modelling. Health Technol Assess. 2007;11(17):1–125.

32. Eborall H, Stone M, Aujla N, Taub N, Davies M, Khunti K. Influences on the uptake of diabetes screening: a qualitative study in primary care. Br J Gen Pract. 2012;62(596):e204–11.

33. Gillies CL, Lambert PC, Abrams KR, Sutton AJ, Cooper NJ, Hsu RT, et al. Different strategies for screening and prevention of type 2 diabetes in adults: cost effectiveness analysis. BMJ. 2008;336(7654):1180–5.

34. Gillett M, Royle P, Snaith A, Scotland G, Poobalan A, Imamura M, et al. Non-pharmacological interventions to reduce the risk of diabetes in people with impaired glucose regulation: a systematic review and economic evaluation. Health Technol Assess. 2012;16(33):1–236.

35. Kahn R, Alperin P, Eddy D, Borch-Johnsen K, Buse J, Feigelman J, et al. Age at initiation and frequency of screening to detect type 2 diabetes: a cost-effectiveness analysis. Lancet. 2010;375(9723):1365–74.

36. Khunti K, Taub N, Gillies C, Abrams K, Hiles S, Webb D, et al. A comparison of screening strategies for impaired glucose tolerance and type 2 diabetes mellitus in a UK community setting: a cost per case analysis. Diabetes Res Clin Pract. 2012;97(3):505–13.

37. Simmons RK, Echouffo-Tcheugui JB, Sharp SJ, Sargeant L, Williams KM, Prevost AT, et al. Screening for type 2 diabetes and population mortality over 10 years (ADDITION-Cambridge): a cluster-randomised controlled trial. Lancet. 2012;380(9855):1741–8.

38. Webb DR, Khunti K, Gray LJ, Srinivasan BT, Farooqi A, Wareham N, et al. Intensive multifactorial intervention improves modelled coronary heart disease risk in screen-detected Type 2 diabetes mellitus: a cluster randomized controlled trial. Diabet Med. 2012;29(4):531–40.

39. Kuo HS, Chang HJ, Chou P, Teng L, Chen TH. A Markov chain model to assess the efficacy of screening for non-insulin dependent diabetes mellitus (NIDDM). Int J Epidemiol. 1999;28:233–40.

40. Rahman M, Simmons RK, Hennings SH, Wareham NJ, Griffin SJ. How much does screening bring forward the diagnosis of type 2 diabetes and reduce complications? Twelve year follow-up of the Ely cohort. Diabetologia. 2012;55(6):1651–9.

Chapter 16
Assessing the Cardiometabolic Risk of Obesity: Importance of Visceral/Ectopic Fat and of the Use of Hypertriglyceridemic Waist

Jean-Pierre Després

Although it is well recognized that overweight/obesity increases the risk of chronic conditions such as hypertension, dyslipidemia, type 2 diabetes, and cardiovascular disease (CVD) [1–4], not every overweight/obese individual will develop these comorbidities [5–8]. For instance, the term "metabolically healthy obese" has even been coined to describe obese patients not characterized by the altered risk factor levels to be expected from their excess body fatness [9–11]. Thus, although clinicians recognize the health risk generally associated with obesity, this heterogeneity of obese patients has left health professionals perplexed for decades. As a consequence, obesity has been considered for a while as a secondary risk factor for CVD behind smoking, hypertension, dyslipidemia, and diabetes.

J.-P. Després, PhD
Department of Kinesiology,
Université Laval, Québec Heart and Lung Institute,
2725, chemin Sainte-Foy, Pavilion Marguerite-D'Youville, Y4146,
Québec City, Québec G1V 4G5, Canada
e-mail: jean-pierre.despres@criucpq.ulaval.ca

D.W. Haslam et al. (eds.), *Controversies in Obesity*,
DOI 10.1007/978-1-4471-2834-2_16,
© Springer-Verlag London 2014

In 1947, a French physician, Jean Vague, was the first to suggest that the complications of obesity were more closely related to body shape than to excess weight [12]. He coined the term "android obesity" to describe the typical body shape characterized by excess upper body fat generally found among men. He suggested that this male pattern of body fat distribution was more dangerous than the female, lower body, adiposity shape (gynoid obesity), which, he proposed, was a rather benign form of obesity. Modern cross-sectional metabolic studies and large prospective studies with hard clinical outcomes that began to be published in the mid-1980s have confirmed Vague's hypothesis in showing that a high proportion of abdominal fat (as crudely estimated by a large waist circumference or by an increased ratio of waist to hip circumference) was predictive of an increased risk of developing type 2 diabetes and cardiovascular outcomes [6–8].

Although these studies really put back at the forefront the concept of regional body fat distribution as clinically relevant information, it is really with the development of imaging technologies such as computed tomography (CT) and magnetic resonance imaging (MRI) that it became possible to systematically assess with great precision the various adipose tissue/fat depots. With CT/MRI, it became rapidly obvious that visceral adipose tissue (which comprises all fat depots in the abdominal cavity) showed a distinct relationship with features of the insulin resistance syndrome [5, 13–24]. For instance, when matched for the amount of total body fat, subjects with a selective excess of visceral adipose tissue were characterized by insulin resistance and related abnormalities [5, 6, 18, 19]. The converse, however, was not true: when two subgroups of individuals matched for visceral adiposity but with high versus low levels of subcutaneous adipose tissue were compared, no substantial difference in their cardiometabolic risk profile was found [18, 19]. Thus, these results clearly show that excess visceral adipose tissue deposition is an important marker of cardiometabolic risk among overweight/obese individuals. Recent prospective studies with imaging measurements of visceral and subcutaneous adipose tissue have clearly confirmed that visceral but not subcutaneous adiposity is related to type 2 diabetes [25, 26].

Although excess visceral adiposity has been associated with a cluster of diabetogenic and atherogenic metabolic abnormalities, the causal relationship between excess visceral adiposity and clinical outcomes has remained uncertain and still debated. While a discussion on the pathophysiology of visceral obesity-related complications is far beyond the scope of this short paper, we have suggested that excess visceral adiposity is largely a marker of the inability of subcutaneous adipose tissue to deal with the energy excess by failing to properly expand through hyperplasia of preadipocytes, leading to accumulation of fat at undesired sites such as the liver, the heart, the skeletal muscle, the kidney, and the pancreas, a phenomenon referred to as ectopic fat deposition [7, 8]. Thus, under this model, excess visceral adipose tissue is a marker of dysfunctional subcutaneous adipose tissue leading to excess ectopic fat. As such, this condition represents the form of overweight/obesity most closely associated with type 2 diabetes and CVD [7, 8].

As excess visceral adipose tissue/ectopic fat cannot be assessed on the basis of the body mass index, a rapid, noninvasive, effective, discriminant, and inexpensive screening tool was needed. In 1994, we suggested that waist circumference was related with visceral adipose tissue deposition, and we later suggested that for a given body mass index, an elevated waist circumference was predictive of an increased deposition of abdominal adipose tissue [27]. However, one remaining problem associated with the waist circumference measurement is that it cannot distinguish subcutaneous from visceral abdominal adiposity. We were therefore very much interested in testing the ability of a simple, widely used, metabolic marker of excess visceral adiposity to improve the discrimination of excess visceral from subcutaneous abdominal adiposity. This was the rationale behind the development of the "hypertriglyceridemic waist" concept, which is defined as the combination of an elevated waistline with a simple plasma marker: fasting triglyceride concentrations [28]. For instance, when the ability of

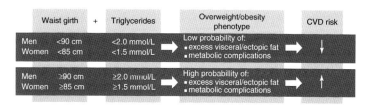

FIGURE 16.1 Use of hypertriglyceridemic waist as a screening tool to identifying individuals likely to be characterized by excess visceral/ectopic fat and related cardiometabolic abnormalities. This model proposes that in the presence of an elevated waist circumference, an elevated fasting triglyceride concentration could represent a marker of the subject's relative inability to accumulate energy surplus in subcutaneous adipose tissue which normally acts as a "metabolic sink" (functional adipose tissue). The hypertriglyceridemic waist phenotype could therefore be considered as a simple marker of "dysfunctional adipose tissue" and of its associated cardiometabolic complications

subcutaneous adipose tissue to clear and store the extra dietary energy gets saturated, the energy must accumulate wherever it can, in the visceral adipose tissue, in the skeletal muscle, in the liver, etc. We have reported a robust relationship between visceral adiposity and liver fat in a large CT imaging cardiometabolic study, the INSPIRE ME IAA study [25]. As a fatty liver is closely related to an overproduction of large VLDL1 particles (which is an attempt of the liver to limit its accumulation of triglycerides), a close relationship is to be expected between excess visceral adiposity, liver fat, and plasma triglyceride levels and, indeed, such association has been found most often [29]. We therefore used waist circumference as a crude index of abdominal adiposity and triglyceride levels as a marker of excess visceral adiposity/liver fat [28]. We then performed sensitivity/specificity analyses to identify the cutoff values which would provide the optimal discrimination of individuals with/without excess visceral adiposity/ectopic fat [28, 30, 31]. These cutoff values are presented in Fig. 16.1. Briefly, whereas absence of hypertriglyceridemic waist was associated with a very low probability (about 10–15 % depending upon the study sample) of being characterized by excess visceral adiposity/ectopic fat and related metabolic abnormalities, hypertriglyceridemic waist was associated with a very high probability (between 75 and 85 %) of being characterized by excess visceral adiposity/ectopic fat, by the constellation of the metabolic abnormalities of insulin resistance and by an increased CHD risk [28, 30, 31]. Since the initial description of this phenotype in 2000, numerous metabolic and prospective studies have shown the added value of using this simple clinical phenotype to rapidly screen for excess visceral adiposity/ectopic fat and related cardiometabolic risk [31–47]. For instance, we tested in the EPIC-Norfolk study the ability of hypertriglyceridemic waist to screen for a constellation of metabolic abnormalities and to discriminate related coronary heart disease (CHD) risk in a large sample of 9,506 men and 12,281 women followed for 9.8 years during which 2,109 cases of incident CHD were recorded [32]. First, very large differences in the baseline cardiometabolic risk profile (blood pressure, HDL cholesterol, apolipoprotein B, C-reactive protein, small and dense LDL) were observed between subjects with versus without hypertriglyceridemic waist, and such difference was observed in both men and women. Secondly, Kaplan-Meier survival curve analyses revealed that hypertriglyceridemic waist was associated with a reduced probability of remaining free from CHD over the follow-up of the study. Thus, results from this large prospective study confirm the relevance of this simple screening tool to identify overweight/obese individuals more likely to be characterized by high levels of visceral adipose tissue/ectopic fat and at increased risk for cardiometabolic outcomes.

In summary, there is emerging evidence that the combination of elevated waist circumference and plasma triglycerides as a phenotype defines a subgroup of patients with a high probability of being characterized by excess levels of visceral adipose tissue/ectopic fat and at increased cardiometabolic risk. Although hypertriglyceridemic waist as a screening tool is simple and cheap, it must be emphasized that it cannot be used as a CVD risk engine nor as a diabetes risk calculator as traditional risk factors must, by all means, be considered in such global risk evaluation. It is rather proposed that the presence/ absence of hypertriglyceridemic waist could nicely complement risk assessment based in classical risk factors performed by current risk engines, which do not consider the additional risk resulting from excess visceral adiposity/ectopic fat.

Acknowledgments Dr. Després is the Scientific Director of the International Chair on Cardiometabolic Risk based at Université Laval. His work has been supported by research grants from the Canadian Institutes of Health Research, the Canadian Diabetes Association, the Heart and Stroke Foundation of Canada, and the Foundation of the Québec Heart and Lung Institute.

References

1. Colditz GA, Willett WC, Rotnitzky A, Manson JE. Weight gain as a risk factor for clinical diabetes mellitus in women. Ann Intern Med. 1995;122:481–6.
2. Willett WC, Manson JE, Stampfer MJ, Colditz GA, Rosner B, Speizer FE, et al. Weight, weight change, and coronary heart disease in women. Risk within the 'normal' weight range. JAMA. 1995;273:461–5.
3. Stamler R, Stamler J, Riedlinger WF, Algera G, Roberts RH. Weight and blood pressure. Findings in hypertension screening of 1 million Americans. JAMA. 1978;240:1607–10.
4. Brown CD, Higgins M, Donato KA, Rohde FC, Garrison R, Obarzanek E, et al. Body mass index and the prevalence of hypertension and dyslipidemia. Obes Res. 2000;8:605–19.
5. Pouliot MC, Després JP, Nadeau A, Moorjani S, Prud'homme D, Lupien PJ, et al. Visceral obesity in men. Associations with glucose tolerance, plasma insulin, and lipoprotein levels. Diabetes. 1992;41:826–34.
6. Després JP, Moorjani S, Lupien PJ, Tremblay A, Nadeau A, Bouchard C. Regional distribution of body fat, plasma lipoproteins, and cardiovascular disease. Arteriosclerosis. 1990;10:497–511.
7. Després JP, Lemieux I. Abdominal obesity and metabolic syndrome. Nature. 2006;444:881–7.
8. Després JP. Body fat distribution and risk of cardiovascular disease: an update. Circulation. 2012;126:1301–13.
9. Primeau V, Coderre L, Karelis AD, Brochu M, Lavoie ME, Messier V, et al. Characterizing the profile of obese patients who are metabolically healthy. Int J Obes (Lond). 2011;35:971–81.
10. Després JP. What is "metabolically healthy obesity"?: from epidemiology to pathophysiological insights. J Clin Endocrinol Metab. 2012; 97:2283–5.

11. Karelis AD, Faraj M, Bastard JP, St-Pierre DH, Brochu M, Prud'homme D, et al. The metabolically healthy but obese individual presents a favorable inflammation profile. J Clin Endocrinol Metab. 2005;90:4145–50.

12. Vague J. Sexual differentiation, a factor affecting the forms of obesity. Presse Med. 1947;30:339–40.

13. Brunzell JD, Hokanson JE. Dyslipidemia of central obesity and insulin resistance. Diabetes Care. 1999;22 Suppl 3:C10–3.

14. Lemieux I, Pascot A, Prud'homme D, Alméras N, Bogaty P, Nadeau A, et al. Elevated C-reactive protein: another component of the atherothrombotic profile of abdominal obesity. Arterioscler Thromb Vasc Biol. 2001;21:961–7.

15. Mertens I, Van der Planken M, Corthouts B, Van Gaal LF. Is visceral adipose tissue a determinant of von Willebrand factor in overweight and obese premenopausal women? Metabolism. 2006;55:650–5.

16. Nieves DJ, Cnop M, Retzlaff B, Walden CE, Brunzell JD, Knopp RH, et al. The atherogenic lipoprotein profile associated with obesity and insulin resistance is largely attributable to intra-abdominal fat. Diabetes. 2003;52:172–9.

17. Pascot A, Lemieux I, Prud'homme D, Tremblay A, Nadeau A, Couillard C, et al. Reduced HDL particle size as an additional feature of the atherogenic dyslipidemia of abdominal obesity. J Lipid Res. 2001;42:2007–14.

18. Ross R, Aru J, Freeman J, Hudson R, Janssen I. Abdominal adiposity and insulin resistance in obese men. Am J Physiol Endocrinol Metab. 2002;282:E657–63.

19. Ross R, Freeman J, Hudson R, Janssen I. Abdominal obesity, muscle composition, and insulin resistance in premenopausal women. J Clin Endocrinol Metab. 2002;87:5044–51.

20. Tchernof A, Lamarche B, Prud'homme D, Nadeau A, Moorjani S, Labrie F, et al. The dense LDL phenotype. Association with plasma lipoprotein levels, visceral obesity, and hyperinsulinemia in men. Diabetes Care. 1996;19:629–37.

21. Björntorp P. Visceral obesity: a "civilization syndrome". Obes Res. 1993; 1:206–22.

22. Boyko EJ, Leonetti DL, Bergstrom RW, Newell-Morris L, Fujimoto WY. Visceral adiposity, fasting plasma insulin, and lipid and lipoprotein levels in Japanese Americans. Int J Obes Relat Metab Disord. 1996;20:801–8.

23. Lebovitz HE, Banerji MA. Point: visceral adiposity is causally related to insulin resistance. Diabetes Care. 2005;28:2322–5.

24. Matsuzawa Y. The role of fat topology in the risk of disease. Int J Obes (Lond). 2008;32 Suppl 7:S83–92.

25. Smith JD, Borel AL, Nazare JA, Haffner SM, Balkau B, Ross R, et al. Visceral adipose tissue indicates the severity of cardiometabolic risk in patients with and without type 2 diabetes: results from the INSPIRE ME IAA study. J Clin Endocrinol Metab. 2012;97:1517–25.

26. Neeland IJ, Turer AT, Ayers CR, Powell-Wiley TM, Vega GL, Farzaneh-Far R, et al. Dysfunctional adiposity and the risk of prediabetes and type 2 diabetes in obese adults. JAMA. 2012;308:1150–9.

27. Pouliot MC, Després JP, Lemieux S, Moorjani S, Bouchard C, Tremblay A, et al. Waist circumference and abdominal sagittal diameter: best simple anthropometric indexes of abdominal visceral adipose tissue accumulation and related cardiovascular risk in men and women. Am J Cardiol. 1994;73:460–8.

28. Lemieux I, Pascot A, Couillard C, Lamarche B, Tchernof A, Alméras N, et al. Hypertriglyceridemic waist. A marker of the atherogenic metabolic triad (hyperinsulinemia, hyperapolipoprotein B, small, dense LDL) in men? Circulation. 2000;102:179–84.

29. Adiels M, Taskinen MR, Packard C, Caslake MJ, Soro-Paavonen A, Westerbacka J, et al. Overproduction of large VLDL particles is driven by increased liver fat content in man. Diabetologia. 2006;49:755–65.

30. Lemieux I, Poirier P, Bergeron J, Alméras N, Lamarche B, Cantin B, et al. Hypertriglyceridemic waist: a useful screening phenotype in preventive cardiology? Can J Cardiol. 2007;23:23B–31.

31. Blackburn P, Lemieux I, Lamarche B, Bergeron J, Perron P, Tremblay G, et al. Type 2 diabetes without the atherogenic metabolic triad does not predict angiographically assessed coronary artery disease in women. Diabetes Care. 2008;31:170–2.

32. Arsenault BJ, Lemieux I, Després JP, Wareham NJ, Kastelein JJ, Khaw KT, et al. The hypertriglyceridemic-waist phenotype and the risk of coronary artery disease: results from the EPIC-Norfolk prospective population study. CMAJ. 2010;182:1427–32.

33. Kahn HS, Valdez R. Metabolic risks identified by the combination of enlarged waist and elevated triacylglycerol concentration. Am J Clin Nutr. 2003;78:928–34.

34. Tanko LB, Bagger YZ, Qin G, Alexandersen P, Larsen PJ, Christiansen C. Enlarged waist combined with elevated triglycerides is a strong predictor of accelerated atherogenesis and related cardiovascular mortality in postmenopausal women. Circulation. 2005;111:1883–90.

35. Blackburn P, Lemieux I, Lamarche B, Bergeron J, Perron P, Tremblay G, et al. Hypertriglyceridemic waist: a simple clinical phenotype associated with coronary artery disease in women. Metabolism. 2012;61:56–64.

36. Egeland GM, Cao Z, Young TK. Hypertriglyceridemic-waist phenotype and glucose intolerance among Canadian Inuit: the International Polar Year Inuit Health Survey for Adults 2007–2008. CMAJ. 2011; 183:E553–8.

37. de Graaf FR, Schuijf JD, Scholte AJ, Djaberi R, van Velzen JE, Roos CJ, et al. Usefulness of hypertriglyceridemic waist phenotype in type 2 diabetes mellitus to predict the presence of coronary artery disease as assessed by computed tomographic coronary angiography. Am J Cardiol. 2010;106:1747–53.

38. Gomez-Huelgas R, Bernal-Lopez MR, Villalobos A, Mancera-Romero J, Baca-Osorio AJ, Jansen S, et al. Hypertriglyceridemic waist: an alternative to the metabolic syndrome? Results of the IMAP Study (multidisciplinary intervention in primary care). Int J Obes (Lond). 2011;35:292–9.

39. Sam S, Haffner S, Davidson MH, D'Agostino Sr RB, Feinstein S, Kondos G, et al. Hypertriglyceridemic waist phenotype predicts increased visceral fat in subjects with type 2 diabetes. Diabetes Care. 2009;32:1916–20.

40. Rogowski O, Shapira I, Steinvil A, Berliner S. Low-grade inflammation in individuals with the hypertriglyceridemic waist phenotype: another feature of the atherogenic dysmetabolism. Metabolism. 2009;58:661–7.

41. St-Pierre J, Lemieux I, Perron P, Brisson D, Santure M, Vohl MC, et al. Relation of the "hypertriglyceridemic waist" phenotype to earlier manifestations of coronary artery disease in patients with glucose intolerance and type 2 diabetes mellitus. Am J Cardiol. 2007;99:369–73.

42. Czernichow S, Bruckert E, Bertrais S, Galan P, Hercberg S, Oppert JM. Hypertriglyceridemic waist and 7.5-year prospective risk of cardiovascular disease in asymptomatic middle-aged men. Int J Obes (Lond). 2007;31:791–6.

43. Bos G, Dekker JM, Heine RJ. Non-HDL cholesterol contributes to the "hypertriglyceridemic waist" as a cardiovascular risk factor: the Hoorn study. Diabetes Care. 2004;27:283–4.

44. LaMonte MJ, Ainsworth BE, DuBose KD, Grandjean PW, Davis PG, Yanowitz FG, et al. The hypertriglyceridemic waist phenotype among women. Atherosclerosis. 2003;171:123–30.

45. Esmaillzadeh A, Mirmiran P, Azizi F. Clustering of metabolic abnormalities in adolescents with the hypertriglyceridemic waist phenotype. Am J Clin Nutr. 2006;83:36–46.

46. Blackburn P, Lamarche B, Couillard C, Pascot A, Bergeron N, Prud'homme D, et al. Postprandial hyperlipidemia: another correlate of the "hypertriglyceridemic waist" phenotype in men. Atherosclerosis. 2003;171:327–36.

47. Lemieux I, Alméras N, Mauriège P, Blanchet C, Dewailly E, Bergeron J, et al. Prevalence of "hypertriglyceridemic waist" in men who participated in the Quebec Health Survey: association with atherogenic and diabetogenic metabolic risk factors. Can J Cardiol. 2002;18:725–32.

Chapter 17
Moving Beyond Scales and Tapes: The Edmonton Obesity Staging System

Arya M. Sharma

Introduction

Although increased body fat can have important implications for health and well-being, the presence of increased body fat alone does not necessarily imply or reliably predict ill health [1, 2]. In addition, anthropometric classifications of obesity based on body mass index (BMI) or waist circumference (WC), while useful in population studies, have clear limitations with regard to guiding clinical decisions in individuals. Thus, although in population studies BMI and WC are reasonable surrogate measures of body and visceral fat, respectively [3, 4], they lack sensitivity and specificity when applied to individuals [5]. People with the same BMI value can have an almost twofold difference in total body fat, while, conversely, individuals with the same amount of total body fat can present with a wide range of BMI [6, 7]. Similarly, there is a large interindividual variation in the amount of visceral fat present in patients with the same WC [4]. This may in part

A.M. Sharma, MD, FRCPC
Department of Medicine, University of Alberta,
Li Ka Shing Building, Rm 1-11687th Avenue and 112th Street,
Edmonton, AB T6G 2E1, Canada
e-mail: amsharm@ualberta.ca

D.W. Haslam et al. (eds.), *Controversies in Obesity*,
DOI 10.1007/978-1-4471-2834-2_17,
© Springer-Verlag London 2014

137

explain the rather flat relationship between anthropometric measures and actual morbidity and mortality found in large epidemiological studies [1, 2]. Evidence suggesting that several factors, including cardiorespiratory fitness, may substantially modify the mortality risk associated with a higher BMI [7], further supporting the notion that BMI alone is insufficient to guide clinical decision-making.

BMI alone provides no measurement of functionality, quality of life, or other prognostic contextual factors that may further characterize clinical risk and guide clinical management. Finally, given the rather poor correlation between anthropometric measures and health, it must be noted that changes in BMI or WC do not necessarily reflect improvement in overall health or functioning. Thus, in an individual, change in obesity class does not necessarily imply improvement or deterioration in overall health or well-being. Conversely, relatively small changes in weight of only 5–10 %, although associated with significant health benefits [8], may not be reflected by changes in obesity class.

The Edmonton Obesity Staging System

In the light of these observations, we recently proposed a classification system for obesity (Edmonton Obesity Staging System, or EOSS) that takes into account physical, mental, and functional limitations associated with excess weight [9] (Table 17.1).

Two recent studies in three large and independent populations have compared EOSS to anthropometric measures like BMI or waist circumference as a predictor of mortality. In the first study, Padwal et al. assessed the EOSS retrospectively using a representative cohort population of overweight and obese patients [10]. In this study, individuals with Class III obesity (after adjustment for metabolic syndrome or waistline) had virtually no increased mortality risk compared to Class II obese individuals (HR 0.9), while individuals with EOSS 2 or 3 had a 4- to 12-fold greater hazard ratio, respectively, compared to individuals with EOSS 0/1. In the second

TABLE 17.1 Clinical and functional staging of obesity

Stage	Description	Management
0	No apparent obesity-related risk factors (e.g., blood pressure, serum lipids, and fasting glucose within normal range), physical symptoms, psychopathology, functional limitations, and/or impairment of well-being	Identification of factors contributing to increased body weight. Counseling to prevent further weight gain through lifestyle measures including healthy eating and increased physical activity
1	Presence of obesity-related subclinical risk factors (e.g., borderline hypertension, impaired fasting glucose, elevated liver enzymes), mild physical symptoms (e.g., dyspnea on moderate exertion, occasional aches and pains, fatigue), mild psychopathology, mild functional limitations, and/or mild impairment of well-being	Investigation for other (non-weight related) contributors to risk factors. More intense lifestyle interventions, including diet and exercise, to prevent further weight gain. Monitoring of risk factors and health status
2	Presence of established obesity-related chronic disease (e.g., hypertension, type 2 diabetes, sleep apnea, osteoarthritis, reflux disease, polycystic ovary syndrome, anxiety disorder), moderate limitations in activities of daily living and/or well-being	Initiation of obesity treatments including considerations of all behavioral, pharmacological, and surgical treatment options. Close monitoring and management of comorbidities as indicated
3	Established end-organ damage such as myocardial infarction, heart failure, diabetic complications, and incapacitating osteoarthritis; significant psychopathology; significant functional limitations; and/or impairment of well-being	More intensive obesity treatment including consideration of all behavioral, pharmacological, and surgical treatment options. Aggressive management of comorbidities as indicated
4	Severe (potentially end stage) disabilities from obesity-related chronic diseases, severe disabling psychopathology, severe functional limitations, and/or severe impairment of well-being	Aggressive obesity management as deemed feasible. Palliative measures including pain management, occupational therapy, and psychosocial support

Adapted from Sharma and Kushner [9]

study by Kuk et al., individuals with EOSS stage 2 or 3 had an increased risk of mortality (HR 1.6–1.7) from all causes compared to normal weight individuals [11], whereas neither EOSS stage 0 nor 1, irrespective of BMI, was associated with increased mortality risk.

Clinical Implications of EOSS

Because EOSS is based on the actual clinical examination of individuals presenting with excess weight, it necessarily gives a far better picture of the health impacts of obesity on that individual than simply measuring BMI or WC. Thus, EOSS is a far better guide for clinical decision-making than any of the anthropometric measures.

This has important implications for the indications of treatments. Thus, for example,

EOSS may help prioritizing patients with increased greater mortality risk (e.g., EOSS stage equal or greater than 2) for treatments such as bariatric surgery, especially in health care systems where access to such procedures is limited. This may also prove a more cost-effective approach as surgical procedures (and probably medications) are more likely to prove cost-effectiveness in individuals with existing comorbidities, who have most to gain from effective obesity management. In contrast, individuals presenting with lower EOSS stages (stages 0–1) may benefit most from supportive management aimed primarily at preventing further weight gain and sustaining current good health rather than a focus on pursuing arbitrary weight-loss goals.

Limitations

Despite potential advantages in guiding clinical practice, EOSS has some limitations. Firstly, it relies on definitions of risk or comorbid conditions that are themselves subject to change. For example, definitions and cutoffs for hypertension, dyslipidemia, or dysglycemia remain in flux. Secondly, clinicians may disagree about whether or not a given risk factor or condition is indeed causally related to or merely aggravated by obesity, and thus whether or not this condition would count towards defining the obesity stage. Thirdly, the proposed system includes subjective parameters such as psychological impact or functional performance where individual patients and clinicians may vary in their judgment of disease severity and thus staging. However, none of these issues are foreign to other classification systems, like the NYHA classification of heart failure or the DSM IV assessment of Axis V global functioning that have worked well in clinical practice to describe and monitor disease states.

Another limitation of the proposed staging system is that when used to merely complement the current anthropometric classification system, it fails to capture weight-related complications that may occur at lower body weights than the current BMI cutoffs. Thus, a male presenting with a BMI of 24 kg/m^2 and a waist circumference of 87 cm, who also has impaired fasting glucose or prehypertension, would not be considered to have stage 1 obesity, because he fails to meet the current anthropometric cutoffs for obesity.

Simply stating the BMI level together with the stage rather than using the current cutoffs of overweight and obesity could remedy this shortcoming. This approach would also help overcome the current limitations imposed by varying anthropometric cutoffs for different ethnic populations. Thus, the patient in the above example would have stage 1 obesity, irrespective of whether he is Caucasian or East Asian. Similarly, the proposed staging system would also have utility in children and adolescents. Indeed, an adaptation of the EOSS system for use in this population is currently underway.

Finally, given the urgent need for a more clinically relevant classification system for obesity, others have proposed similar systems based on presence of relevant comorbidities [12]. To date no direct comparisons between EOSS and such systems have been undertaken.

Current Use

Despite these limitations, EOSS has begun finding its way into clinical practice. Assessing obesity stage is part of the recommended workup of the Assess phase of the 5As of Obesity Management framework proposed by the Canadian Obesity Network [13]. EOSS is currently also being discussed as a basis for setting goals for public health interventions [14] and defining outcomes in clinical trials [15].

Summary

EOSS represents a simple clinical staging framework that provides an indication of obesity-related disease extent and severity. In addition, it is a better predictor of mortality than current anthropometric measures of obesity such as BMI or WC. Thus, EOSS not only has the potential to enhance clinical decision-making but could also serve as a useful tool for researchers, payers, and policy makers to better define the impact of excess body fat on health and well-being.

References

1. Flegal KM, Graubard BI, Williamson DF, Gail MH. Cause-specific excess deaths associated with underweight, overweight, and obesity. JAMA. 2007;298:2028–37.
2. Pischon T, Boeing H, Hoffmann K, Bergmann M, Schulze MB, Overvad K, et al. General and abdominal adiposity and risk of death in Europe. N Engl J Med. 2008;359:2105–20.
3. Lean MEJ, Han TS, Deurenberg P. Predicting body composition by densitometry from simple anthropometric measurements. Am J Clin Nutr. 1996;63:4–14.
4. Rankinen T, Kim SY, Pérusse L, Després JP, Bouchard C. The prediction of abdominal visceral fat level from body composition and anthropometry: ROC analysis. Int J Obes Relat Metab Disord. 1999;23:801–9.
5. Wellens RI, Roche AF, Khamis HJ, Jackson AS, Pollock ML, Siervogel RM. Relationships between body mass index and body composition. Obes Res. 1996;4:35–44.

6. Gallagher D, Heymsfield SB, Heo M, Jebb SA, Murgatroyd PR, Sakamoto Y. Healthy percentage body fat ranges: an approach for developing guidelines based on body mass index. Am J Clin Nutr. 2000;72:694–701.
7. Sui X, LaMonte MJ, Laditka JN, Hardin JW, Chase N, Hooker SP, Blair SN. Cardiorespiratory fitness and adiposity as mortality predictors in older adults. JAMA. 2007;298:2507–16.
8. World Health Organization. Report of a WHO consultation on obesity. Obesity: preventing and managing the global epidemic. Geneva: World Health Organization; 1998.
9. Sharma AM, Kushner RF. A proposed clinical staging system for obesity. Int J Obes. 2009;33:289–95.
10. Padwal RS, Pajewski NM, Allison DB, Sharma AM. Using the edmonton obesity staging system to predict mortality in a population-representative cohort of people with overweight and obesity. CMAJ. 2011;183:E1059–66.
11. Kuk JL, Ardern CI, Church TS, Sharma AM, Padwal R, Sui X, et al. Edmonton obesity staging system: association with weight history and mortality risk. Appl Physiol Nutr Metab. 2011;36:570–6.
12. Aasheim ET, Aylwin SJB, Radhakrishnan ST, Sood AS, Jovanovic A, Olbers T, le Roux CW. Assessment of obesity beyond body mass index to determine benefit of treatment. Clin Obes. 2011;1:77–84.
13. Vallis M, Piccinini-Vallis H, Sharma AM, Freedhoff Y. Modified 5 as minimal intervention for obesity counseling in primary care. Can Fam Physician. 2013;59:27–31.
14. Northern health position on health, weight and obesity: an integrated population health Approach 2012. Accessed at: http://www.northernhealth.ca/Portals/0/About/PositionPapers/documents/HealthWtObesityPosition_20120730_WEB.pdf.
15. Ferguson C, David S, Divine L, Kahan S, Gallagher C, Gooding M, Markell P. Obesity drug outcome measures: a consensus report of considerations regarding pharmacologic intervention. The George Washington University, School of Public Health and Health Services 2012. Accessed at: http://sphhs.gwu.edu/releases/obesitydrugmeasures.pdf.

Chapter 18
Obstructive Sleep Apnea

Bertrand R. de Silva

Obstructive sleep apnea (OSA) is the pathologic narrowing of the airway during sleep that causes the brain to repetitively arouse. The increased incidence of OSA [1] is due to the rising rates of obesity and improved recognition of this condition in both males [2] (25 %) and females (10 %) with age [3, 4]. OSA is not confined to the extreme of age and is present in young children due to enlarged tonsils and adolescents due to inherited and acquired (by orthodontic treatment teeth extraction) craniofacial abnormalities [5]. Unfortunately, only a minority of patients with OSA have been evaluated [6]. Subtle cases of OSA are not easily recognized at an early stage of disease evolution [7], especially in females [8–10], and lead to the frequent misinterpretation of OSA as it masquerades as attention deficit disorder (ADD), chronic fatigue syndrome, fibromyalgia, Epstein–Barr virus (EBV) infection, hormonal deficiency, depression, and anxiety. It is the absence of education and training in sleep medicine at preclinical, clinical, and postgraduate levels that accounts for misdiagnosis [11].

The states of wakefulness (sympathetic) and sleep (parasympathetic) are a consequence of the normal physiologic

B.R. de Silva, MBBS, FCCP, DABSM
2133 west Chapman Avenue,
Suite H, Orange, California 92868, USA
e-mail: srilankan1@aol.com

D.W. Haslam et al. (eds.), *Controversies in Obesity*,
DOI 10.1007/978-1-4471-2834-2_18,
© Springer-Verlag London 2014

oscillation of the autonomic nervous system and hormonal secretion. If OSA is superimposed on the normal quiescent parasympathetic stage of sleep, it cyclically increases sympathetic tone by initiating adrenaline and cortisol release with resultant hypertension [12] and tachycardia that is accompanied by the episodes of oxygen desaturation. The long-term adverse consequences of OSA are directly linked to the protective mechanisms of the fight-or-flight reaction to the apneic events. Night sweats, anxiety and depression, disturbing and violent pursuit dreams, post-traumatic stress disorder (PTSD), episodes of wakefulness after sleep onset (WASO), insomnia, incessant nocturia (due to atrial natriuretic factor release), loud snoring, snorts and gasps, witnessed apneas, gastroesophageal reflux disease (GERD), non-restorative sleep, symptoms of excessive daytime sleepiness (EDS), myocardial infarction (MI), cardiac arrhythmias, exacerbations of chronic obstructive airways disease (COPD), congestive heart failure (CHF) and angina, atrial fibrillation, cardiomyopathy and cor pulmonale, erectile dysfunction (ED) due to low testosterone secretion from rapid eye movement (REM) sleep deprivation, loss of short-term memory, morning headache, marital discord, excessive alcohol [5, 13, 14] and stimulant consumption, unexplained weight gain, and adaptation of lifestyle and dietary intake to chronic sleepiness and fatigue may result. Comorbid illness in the form of diabetes [14], uncontrolled hypertension, stroke [15], and increased risk of motor vehicle accidents (MVA) are common. Sleep apnea is the greatest stress test that a body can be put through and often patients do not survive, leading to four-to sixfold increase in the rates of early morning deaths [15].

Previously the diagnosis of OSA by polysomnography (PSG) required cumbersome expensive equipment with a dedicated location under strict clinical conditions for the sensors to measure the necessary physiologic parameters. Now with the pathophysiology clearly defined, it is apparent that the majority of suspected patients without moderate comorbidities (85 %) can move from the laboratory to home sleep tests (HST). Improved technology and data gathering have reduced complexity, increased access, and reduced the cost. The wide availability of continuous positive airway pressure (CPAP) machines that are auto-titrating has further reduced complexity and improved compliance with treatment. The threshold for treatment has decreased with an appreciation that not all OSA manifests with clearly definable apneas and hypopneas. Treatment trials with CPAP for patients with symptoms and multiple comorbidities without a qualifying apnea hypopnea index (AHI) for proof of concept seem appropriate. "Does all sleep apnea need to be treated?" is a question frequently asked, and the response should be affirmative to achieve an improvement in both the quality and quantity of life. With evolution in technology, empiric treatment may be instituted, looking for clinical improvement, and only treatment failures will be referred for sleep physician evaluation and sleep studies. Attempts by the dental profession to encroach upon the medical management of sleep apnea with expensive mandibular advancement devices (MAD) and mandibular retaining devices (MRD) dental devices that do not address all levels of obstruction and are a poor substitute for CPAP should be strenuously resisted by sleep physicians. CPAP should remain the primary modality of treatment offered to all patients. MRD and MAD should be treatments considered only for snoring without apnea or in CPAP-intolerant patients with mild sleep apnea only. The adoption of any other treatment algorithm would constitute malpractice.

OSA is the most underdiagnosed and untreated condition in all of medicine. The incidence and prevalence of OSA exceeds the sum of cardiac and pulmonary disease. It is so prevalent that it may be considered to be normal. It is a consequence of the evolution of the human species and the quest for an upright stance and vocalization that has resulted in the hollow tube of the oropharynx becoming collapsible. Changes in the lifestyle, nutrition, increased life expectancy, and obesity rates of industrialized countries have further compounded the instability of this airway. The use of mind- and mood-altering drugs, including alcohol, sedatives, narcotics, and hypnotics, has further increased the rates of OSA. There is a need for the improved education of the primary doctor in the pathophysiologic mechanisms of OSA and for a greater appreciation of the different guises that OSA adopts. Public awareness programs should be instituted. The economics of under- and misdiagnosed OSA are enormous, including lost earnings as a result of disability and premature death. The Medicare requirement for a sleep lab not to provide treatment has also caused the sleep physicians to be involved in the diagnosis but to be divorced from the treatment. The burden of initiating, problem solving, and monitoring treatment has thus fallen on the poorly trained primary care physician. The general poor outcomes of the process of diagnosis and CPAP treatment adherence (47–53 %) have further compounded the reluctance of health care providers to refer for diagnostic evaluation. The realization that OSA represents a vast untapped pool of potential cost saving in an environment of economic contraction should spur the diagnosis and treatment. With enactment of new health care laws and formation of accountability care organizations (ACO), OSA represents an area where early diagnosis and preventative care would reduce medication and hospitalization costs.

References

1. Young T, Peppard PE, Gottlieb DJ. Epidemiology of obstructive sleep apnea: a population health perspective. Am J Respir Crit Care Med. 2002;165(9):1217–39.
2. Bixler EO, Vgontzas AN, Ten Have T, Tyson K, Kales A. Effects of age on sleep apnea in men: I. Prevalence and severity. Am J Respir Crit Care Med. 1998;157:144–8.
3. Young T, Palta M, Dempsey J, Skatrud J, Weber S, Badr S. The occurrence of sleep-disordered breathing among middle-aged adults. N Engl J Med. 1993;328:1230–5.
4. Malhotra A, Huang Y, Fogel R, Lazic S, Pillar G, Jakab M, Kikinis R, White DP. Aging influences on pharyngeal anatomy and physiology: the predisposition to pharyngeal collapse. Am J Med. 2006;119:72.e9–14.
5. Miles PG, Vig PS, Weyant RJ, Forrest TD, Rockette Jr HE. Craniofacial structure and obstructive sleep apnea syndrome–a qualitative analysis and meta-analysis of the literature. Am J Orthod Dentofacial Orthop. 1996;109:163–72.

6. Bixler EO, Vgontzas AN, Lin HM, Ten Have T, Rein J, Vela-Bueno A, Kales A. Prevalence of sleep-disordered breathing in women: effects of gender. Am J Respir Crit Care Med. 2001;163:608–13.

7. Kapur V, Strohl KP, Redline S, Iber C, O'Connor G, Nieto J. Underdiagnosis of sleep apnea syndrome in US communities. Sleep Breath. 2002;6:49–54.

8. Fogel RB, Malhotra A, White DP. Sleep. 2: pathophysiology of obstructive sleep apnoea/hypopnoea syndrome. Thorax. 2004;59:159–63.

9. Shepertycky MR, Banno K, Kryger MH. Differences between men and women in the clinical presentation of patients diagnosed with obstructive sleep apnea syndrome. Sleep. 2005;28:309–14.

10. Jordan AS, McEvoy RD. Gender differences in sleep apnea: epidemiology, clinical presentation and pathogenic mechanisms. Sleep Med Rev. 2003;7:377–89.

11. Levitzky MG. Using the pathophysiology of obstructive sleep apnea to teach cardiopulmonary integration. Adv Physiol Educ. 2008;32:196–202.

12. Peppard PE, Young T, Palta M, Skatrud J. Prospective study of the association between sleep-disordered breathing and hypertension. N Engl J Med. 2000;342:1378–84.

13. Peppard PE, Austin D, Brown RL. Association of alcohol consumption and sleep disordered breathing in men and women. J Clin Sleep Med. 2007;3:265–70.

14. Reichmuth KJ, Austin D, Skatrud JB, Young T. Association of sleep apnea and type II diabetes: a population-based study. Am J Respir Crit Care Med. 2005;172:1590–5.

15. Yaggi HK, Concato J, Kernan WN, Lichtman JH, Brass LM, Mohsenin V. Obstructive sleep apnea as a risk factor for stroke and death. N Engl J Med. 2005;353:2034–41.

Chapter 19
Obesity and the Heart Disease Patient: Controversies Abound

Henry J. Purcell

Introduction

If we define a controversy as "a prolonged dispute, debate or contention, concerning a matter of opinion," then there is no shortage of controversy relating to obesity and the coronary heart disease (CHD) patient. In simple terms, obese people are 80 times more likely to develop type 2 diabetes, and 75 % or more of patients with diabetes die of cardiovascular causes, often prematurely [1]. Indeed, "overwhelming evidence supports the importance of obesity in the pathogenesis and progression of cardiovascular disease" [2]. However, obesity rates are rapidly increasing worldwide, and in the UK they are the highest in Europe. In England, rates have increased faster than most OECD countries. Figures from the 2012 *Health Survey for England* [3] show that in 2010, just over a quarter of adults (26 % of both men and women) were obese and 42 % of men and 32 % of women were overweight.

The incidence of CHD has declined appreciably, by almost two-thirds, among men in the UK over the last 25 years.

H.J. Purcell, MB, PhD
Department of Cardiology, Royal Brompton Hospital,
Sydney Street, London SW3 6NP, UK
e-mail: henry.purcell@rbht.nhs.uk

D.W. Haslam et al. (eds.), *Controversies in Obesity*,
DOI 10.1007/978-1-4471-2834-2_19,
© Springer-Verlag London 2014

About half of the decline can be accounted for by favorable trends in risk factor control, e.g., reductions in blood pressure and smoking. Frustratingly, however, this decline is being curbed by the negative contribution of the population rise in mean body mass index (BMI), provoking a plea that the problem needs "urgent attention" [4].

What Is Obesity?

BMI has been the linchpin of weight measurement, and there is considerable evidence that BMI is unable to distinguish between people with excess adipose tissue and those with high muscle mass. Thus, using BMI may result in misclassification of risk. As BMI cannot always discriminate between those people who are at high risk of developing cardiovascular disease, other parameters, including waist circumference (WC) – a proxy for visceral (abdominal) adiposity – waist to hip ratio, and measures of body fat, along with a set of metabolic markers, may provide better "at risk" data than more conventional measures [5, 6]. The metabolic syndrome, which tends to have evolving diagnostic criteria, is characterized by a clustering of risk markers such as central adiposity, insulin resistance, raised blood pressure, dyslipidemia, and a pro-inflammatory-prothrombotic state, and it defines a condition with high cardiovascular risk. It is suggested that only a small amount of steady weight loss of between 10 and 15 % of initial body weight is adequate to improve the metabolic-syndrome-associated risk factors and progression to type 2 diabetes [7].

In contrast, somewhat controversially, Swiss workers have proposed BMI as a valuable alternative to cholesterol in cardiovascular disease risk prediction models [8], although this needs to be validated in other populations.

While BMI continues to be used clinically, evidence suggests that this may be misleading among two groups in particular, children [9] and South Asians [10].

Atherosclerosis begins in early life. Although BMI may be regarded as a reliable indicator of body fatness for most children and teens, it may become unreliable in children who are short and muscular, for example, and who may be labeled incorrectly as being overweight. In contrast, recent research from the UK suggests that there are inconsistencies between different measures among children that may mean that obesity levels in children are actually underestimated, which in turn gives "mixed public health messages" [9].

South Asian communities, which represent one fifth of the global population, are prone to developing CHD at a younger age, often before the age of 40 years in males [10]. As shown in the INTERHEART study [11], conventional cardiovascular risk factors account for the majority of attributable risk for myocardial infarction in all ethnic groups, including South Asians. However, South Asians have increased abdominal fat and greater insulin resistance at similar levels of BMI, which suggest that reliance on BMI alone may underestimate true risk in this population. Kumar et al. [12] suggest that there is an urgent need to establish appropriate thresholds for waist circumference and whether lower treatment thresholds are warranted among British South Asians.

Imaging and Inflammation

Adipose tissue is now recognized as an endocrine/paracrine organ that produces a variety of inflammatory cytokines (e.g., interlukin-6 [IL-6]) as well as anti-inflammatory adipokines (e.g., adiponectin), which are modulators of atherosclerosis. Whether analyzing the overall inflammatory activity of adipose tissue, with a view to designing inhibitors of inflammatory and atherogenesis activity, will be clinically worthwhile remains to be shown. However it has fuelled enthusiasm to image abdominal fat, initially using computed tomography (CT), but more recently the focus is on epicardial/pericardial fat, viewed without ionizing radiation techniques such as magnetic resonance imaging (MRI) and echocardiography. Adipose tissue surrounds approximately 80 % of the surface area of the human heart, and it increases in the obese. Obesity increases the likelihood of developing atrial fibrillation (AF). Pericardial fat is associated with the presence and severity of AF, and a local pathogenic effect of pericardial fat on the atria, which may promote arrhythmogenesis, has recently been proposed [13]. While using, in this particular case, MRI to image epicardial fat, the utility and cost-effectiveness of such imaging in clinical care has yet to be proven.

The Obesity Paradox

Perhaps one of the most controversial of all observations is the "obesity" paradox. Typically, obesity confers increased risk of cardiovascular and coronary heart disease; paradoxically, however, overweight and obese individuals with established CVD have a better prognosis compared with non-overweight and nonobese individuals [2]. Although counterintuitive, and unexplained, the concept of the paradox has recently been strengthened by data from a large Swedish registry showing a U-shaped relationship between BMI and mortality in acute coronary syndrome (ACS) patients with the nadir among overweight/obese patients and underweight and normal-weight individuals having the highest risk [14].

Perhaps the greatest controversial, dietary challenge ahead to improve public health will be to manipulate conditions, whereby energy input = energy output [15].

Conclusion

Obesity rates are rising and associated with premature cardiovascular and other diseases. Obesity is often defined on measures of BMI, which has limitations, especially when used as a metric among children and within certain populations such as South Asians. There is enthusiasm for measuring visceral fat and imaging it noninvasively, but the benefits of such studies may have more academic than clinical merit. Finally of all the controversies in obesity, the "obesity paradox" remains one of the most elusive to explain.

References

1. Diabetes & obesity: a heavy burden. Report from Diabetes UK. 2005;03:3–17.
2. Lavie CJ, Milani MD, Ventura HO. Obesity and cardiovascular disease. Risk factor, paradox, and impact of weight loss. J Am Coll Cardiol. 2009;53:1925–32.
3. Statistics on obesity, physical activity, and diet: England. The NHS Information Centre. 2012. Available at www.ic.nhs.uk/pubs/opad12.
4. Hardoon SL, Morris RW, Whincup PH, Shipley MJ, Britton AR, Masset G, et al. Rising adiposity curbing decline in the incidence of myocardial infarction: 20-year follow-up of British men and women in the Whitehall II cohort. Eur Heart J. 2012;33:478–85.
5. Lavie CJ, De Schutter A, Patel DA, Romero-Corral A, Artham SM, Milani RV. Body composition and survival in stable coronary heart disease. Impact of lean mass index and body fat in the "obesity paradox". J Am Coll Cardiol. 2012;60(15):1374–80.
6. Poirier P. Cardiologists and abdominal obesity: lost in translation? Heart. 2009;95:1033–5.
7. Morrell J, Fox KAA. Prevalence of abdominal obesity in primary care: the IDEA UK study. Int J Clin Pract. 2009;63:1301–7.
8. Faeh D, Braun J, Bopp M. Body mass index vs cholesterol in cardiovascular disease risk prediction models. (Research letter). Arch Intern Med. 2012;172(22):1766–8.
9. Griffiths C, Gately P, Marchant PR, Cooke CB. Cross-sectional comparisons of BMI and waist circumference in British children: mixed public health messages. Obesity. 2012;20:1258–60.
10. Gupta M, Singh N, Verma S. South Asians and cardiovascular risk. What clinicians should know. Circulation. 2006;113:e924–9.
11. Yusuf S, Hawken S, Ounpuu S, Dans T, Avezum A, Lanas F, INTERHEART Study Investigators, et al. Effect of potentially modifiable risk factors associated with myocardial infarction in 52 countries (the INTERHEART study): case–control study. Lancet. 2004;364:937–52.
12. Kumar S, Hanif W, Zaman MJ, Sattar N, Patel K, Khunti K. Lower thresholds for diagnosis and management of obesity in British South Asians. Int J Clin Pract. 2011;65:375–9.
13. Wong CX, Abed HS, Molaee P, Nelson AJ, Brooks AG, Sharma G, et al. Pericardial fat is associated with atrial fibrillation severity and ablation outcome. J Am Coll Cardiol. 2011;57:1745–51.
14. Angeras O, Albertsson P, Karason K, Råmunddal T, Matejka G, James S, et al. Evidence for obesity paradox in patients with acute coronary syndromes:a report from the Swedish Coronary Angiography and Angioplasty Registry. Eur Heart J. 2013;34(5):345–53.
15. Purcell H, Daly C, Day C, Ziso B, Wilding J. Chapter 1. Chronic non-communicable diseases: adding weight to evidence. In: Chronic non-communicable diseases: weight of evidence for an ounce of prevention. London: NSHI Publishers; 2012. p. 1–11.

Chapter 20
Obesity, Diabetes, and Dental Health: Relationship and Management

Rajesh Chauhan

Obesity and Periodontal Disease

In addition to the accepted complications of diabetes that include macrovascular or microvascular involvement, evidence has emerged of a further complication – periodontal disease (PD) – affecting the tissues surrounding and supporting the teeth [1–3]. Studies suggest that diabetes is often reported in individuals with increased prevalence and severity of periodontal destruction [4]. Indeed, people with diabetes are twice as likely to develop PD compared with those in the general population [5, 6]. However, interpretation of the data has not always been straightforward, due to variations in classification and study design [2]. Individuals with diabetes and retinopathy are up to five times more likely to have advanced PD compared with those without retinal involvement [1]. Furthermore, PD is a strong predictor of mortality

R. Chauhan, BDS (London),
FDSRCS (England), FFDRCS (Ireland)
Watton Place Clinic, 60 High Street,
Watton at Stone, Hertfordshire SG14 3SY, UK
e-mail: dentalsurgery@wattonplaceclinic.com

D.W. Haslam et al. (eds.), *Controversies in Obesity*,
DOI 10.1007/978-1-4471-2834-2_20,
© Springer-Verlag London 2014

risk from cardiovascular and renal complications. In Pima Indian populations with type 2 diabetes and severe PD, deaths from ischemic heart disease were 2.3-fold and 8.5-fold higher, respectively, from diabetic nephropathy, compared with those with no or mild/moderate (combined) PD [7]. Thus, early identification of diabetes is essential and suggests a fundamental role for the dental practitioner in multidisciplinary team.

Dental Health and Disease

The most prevalent dental disorders are erosion, caries, and PD [8].

Dental erosion is a progressive deterioration of the hard tissue by acids, with no bacterial or sugar involvement and is not infectious (Fig. 20.1). Erosion may be caused by acids produced intrinsically in the body, extrinsically from the diet, occupational environment, eating disorders, or dietary practices involving frequent intake of acidic foods and beverages – all may impair the integrity of the tooth. The etiology of deterioration differs according to diet and nutrition [8].

Dental caries is caused by the decalcification of the tooth enamel by oral bacteria as carbohydrates are metabolized into acids (Fig. 20.2), often as a response to regular or overconsumption of sugar-sweetened beverages (SSBs) and food. Cariogenesis occurs with a loss of mineral (demineralization) when plaque pH drops below 5.5, and redeposition (remineralization) occurs when pH rises. Fluoride increases pH by 0.5 units thereby exerting its protective effect. Whether a lesion develops relies on the fine balance between demineralization and remineralization – the latter being significantly slower than the former [8].

PD, an infectious oral condition affecting the supporting structures of the teeth, occurs in response to bacterial products found in plaque. Bacteria are required, but not sufficient, for disease initiation [9]. Studies show that a persistent host inflammatory response is necessary before the soft and mineralized periodontal tissues are eroded [9, 10].

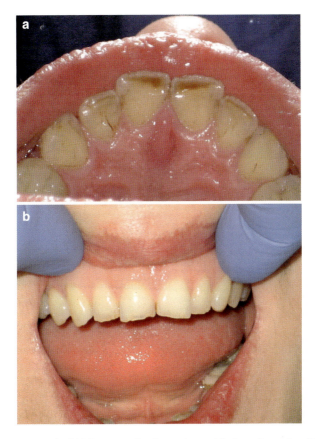

FIGURE 20.1 (**a**, **b**) Photograph of a patient with dental erosion. This is caused by the progression deterioration of the hard tissue by acids and is not infectious (Courtesy of Dr. Rajesh Chauhan)

PD includes gingivitis and periodontitis (Fig. 20.3). Gingivitis occurs where inflamed tissues in the gum are associated with a tooth that is not currently losing attachment or bone, or that has reduced periodontal support. This is commonly associated with plaque buildup, which if left untreated, can lead to periodontitis. Periodontitis is a more advanced form of disease, caused when specific microorganisms colonize, triggering progressive destruction of the periodontal

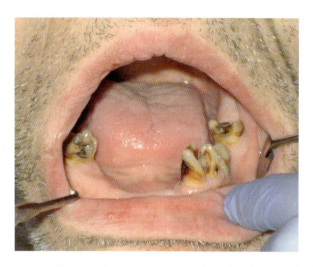

Figure 20.2 Photograph of a patient with dental caries. Dissolution of the teeth is caused by the acids formed during the metabolism of dietary carbohydrates by bacteria and is infectious (Courtesy of Dr. Rajesh Chauhan)

ligament and alveolar bone, with pocket formation or recession around diseased teeth (or both) [1]. This multifactorial process includes microbial challenge alongside other genetic, environmental, and acquired risk factors. The destructive tissue changes observed clinically are as a result of the host's inflammatory response.

Type 2 diabetes is commonly linked to obesity, which contributes to insulin resistance by the elevation of circulating free fatty acids that inhibit glucose update, glycogen synthesis, and glycolysis [11]. Adipose tissue produces a range of adipocytokines, whose levels are altered in people with diabetes; these changes appear to stimulate pathogenic processes associated with metabolic and cardiovascular disease [12]. Metabolic control is important in diabetes, not only to reduce the risk of developing complications, but because individuals are more susceptible to infectious disease than those without – by a two- to fivefold risk for periodontitis [13]. Thus, a complex bidirectional relationship exists between type 2 diabetes

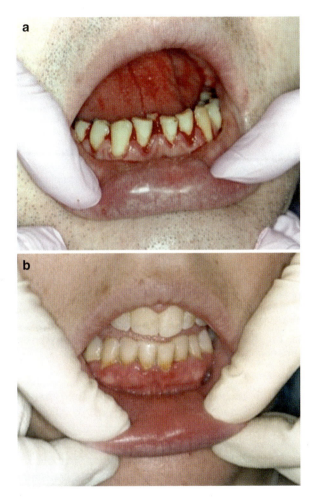

FIGURE 20.3 (**a**) Photograph of a patient with gingivitis and underlying PD. If gingivitis were treated at this stage, bone loss due to PD would be minimal (Courtesy of Dr. Rajesh Chauhan). (**b**) Photograph of a patient with PD. Accompanying radiographs (not shown) would indicate attachment and bone loss (Courtesy of Dr. Rajesh Chauhan)

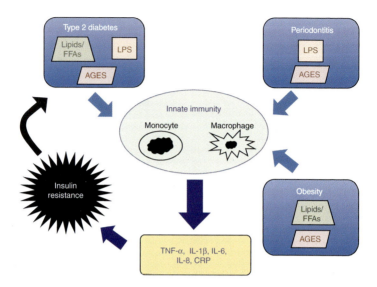

FIGURE 20.4 Common mediators and proinflammatory markers of innate immunity in type 2 diabetes, periodontitis, and obesity. Inappropriate secretion of such molecules may perpetuate an inflammatory state, worsening diabetes and leading to the destruction of periodontal tissue (Adapted from Tunes et al. [11])

and PD, with each being a risk factor for the other. Type 2 diabetes, obesity, and periodontitis are linked by inflammation – triggered systemically by cytokines from adipose tissue and locally by an infected gum [14]. Activation of the innate immune system produces a cytokine-induced response, resulting in low-grade inflammation and increased concentrations of various acute-phase markers and proinflammatory cytokines (Fig. 20.4) [11]. Increased levels of tumor necrosis factor (TNF)-α, interleukin (IL)-1β, IL-6, and IL-8 have been found in gingival fluid, suggesting an important role in the inflammatory process [11]. TNF-α is key in the pathogenesis of periodontitis and increased concentrations can cause insulin resistance [3]. Chronic periodontal infections can initiate or perpetuate insulin resistance and glycemia in a similar way to obesity; locally produced cytokines move into the systemic

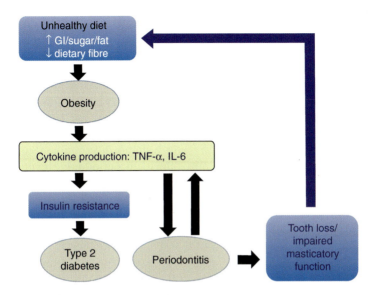

FIGURE 20.5 Association between periodontitis and type 2 diabetes and/or obesity implies that periodontitis and obesity are related to each other, and that this relationship may result in a vicious cycle (Adapted from Nagasawa et al. [16])

circulation, enhancing the immune response and exacerbating an elevated inflammatory state [11, 15], which can worsen diabetes (Fig. 20.5). The formation of advanced end products – central to diabetes complications – also occurs in the periodontium [3]. Thus, inappropriate cytokine production due to obesity-related inflammation indicates an impaired immune response that can lead to periodontitis.

Improving Glycemia

Poor glycemic control is associated with an increased risk of developing diabetes complications [14]. The link between periodontitis and diabetes is also more pronounced with reduced glycemic control [17], and the extent is likely to be a key factor in determining risk. In a large American epidemiological study, adults with poorly controlled diabetes had a 2.9-fold increased risk for periodontitis compared with those without; individuals with well-controlled diabetes had no significant increase in risk [17].

Periodontal treatment that removes microbial biofilm may reduce levels of circulating TNF-α in people with PD, improving diabetes control through the reduction of insulin resistance and restoring insulin sensitivity [15]. Studies suggest that scaling and root planing with systemic doxycycline therapy are associated with improvement in periodontal health and significant improvement in glycemic control (measured by HbA1c) [18, 19]. These studies are notoriously difficult to interpret, however, as other glucose-lowering interventions may have confounded the results, or individuals decided to improve both glycemic control and periodontal health simultaneously. Also, some participants demonstrate marked improvements in glycemia after periodontal intervention, while others exhibit no change after similar regimens [20]. Consequently, the exact extent of the bidirectional link has still to be decided, and further research is required in a cohort population with similar baseline levels of PD and glycemia.

Dental Health and the Future

Sugar and poor dental health are intrinsically linked and may contribute to an elevated inflammatory state. It is also likely that caries and obesity are interrelated [21] and certainly coexist in children, particularly those of low socioeconomic status [22]. Sugar, refined carbohydrates, and, in particular, SSB impact upon dental health and can lead to obesity [23, 24]. Overconsumption of SSB (e.g., carbonated/powdered fruit and sports drinks, sweetened fruit juices), and to a lesser extent 100 % juice, is also associated with increased caries risk [25].

Obesity and type 2 diabetes are two of the most concerning health-care challenges we face today. Dental practitioners are ideally placed to offer obesity prevention and management advice and education, through recognition of the relationship between oral health and diet. To reduce the number of people affected by obesity, diabetes, and its complications (including PD), health-care professionals will need to proactively increase awareness of the risks, to improve self-management and provide a more effective and integrated health-care solution.

References

1. Löe H. Periodontal disease. The sixth complication of diabetes mellitus. Diabetes Care. 1993;16(1):329–34.
2. Mealey BL. Periodontal disease and diabetes: a two-way street. J Am Dent Assoc. 2006;137:26S–31.
3. Mealey BL, Ocampo GL. Diabetes mellitus and periodontal disease. Periodontol 2000. 2007;44:127–53.
4. Lakschevitz F, Aboodi G, Tenenbaum H, Glogauer M. Diabetes and periodontal diabetes and periodontal diseases: interplay and links. Curr Diabetes Rev. 2011;7(6):433–9.
5. Nelson RG, Shlossman M, Budding LM, Pettitt DJ, Saad MF, Genco RJ, et al. Periodontal disease and NIDDM in Pima Indians. Diabetes Care. 1990;13:836–40.
6. Firatli E. The relationship between clinical periodontal status and insulin-dependent diabetes mellitus. Results after 5 years. J Periodontol. 1997;68:136–40.
7. Saremi A, Nelson RG, Tulloch-Reid M, Hanson RL, Sievers ML, Taylor GW, et al. Periodontal disease and mortality in type 2 diabetes. Diabetes Care. 2005;28:27–32.
8. Touger-Decker R, van Loveren C. Sugars and dental caries. Am J Clin Nutr. 2003;78(Suppl):881S–92.
9. Graves D. Cytokines that promote periodontal tissue destruction. J Periodontol. 2008;79(8 Suppl):1585S–91.
10. Liu YC, Lerner UH, Teng YT. Cytokine responses against periodontal infection: protective and destructive roles. Periodontol 2000. 2000;2010(52):163–206.
11. Tunes SR, Foss-Freitas MC, Nogueira-Filho Gda R. Impact of periodontitis on the diabetes-related inflammatory status. J Can Dent Assoc. 2010;76:a35.
12. Bays H, Mandarino L, DeFronzo R. Role of the adipocyte, free fatty acids, and ectopic fat in pathogenesis of type 2 diabetes mellitus: peroxisomal proliferator-activated receptor agonists provide a rational therapeutic approach. J Clin Endocrinol Metab. 2004;89:463–78.
13. UK Prospective Diabetes Study (UKPDS) Group. Intensive blood-glucose control with sulphonylureas or insulin compared with conventional treatment and risk of complications in patients with type 2 diabetes (UKPDS 33). Lancet. 1998;352(9131):837–53.

14. UK Prospective Diabetes Study 6. Complications in newly diagnosed type 2 diabetic patients and their association with different clinical and biochemical risk factors. Diabetes Res. 1990;13(1):1–11.
15. Mealey BL, Rose LF. Diabetes mellitus and inflammatory periodontal diseases. Curr Opin Endocrinol Diabetes Obes. 2008;15(2):135–41.
16. Nagasawa T, Noda M, Katagiri S, Takaichi M, Takahashi Y, Wara-Aswapati N, et al. Relationship between periodontitis and diabetes-importance of a clinical study to prove the vicious cycle. Intern Med. 2010;49:881–5.
17. Tsai C, Hayes C, Taylor GW. Glycemic control of type 2 diabetes and severe periodontal disease in the US adult population. Community Dent Oral Epidemiol. 2002;30:182–92.
18. Grossi SG, Skrepcinski FB, DeCaro T, Zambon JJ, Cummins D, Genco RJ, et al. Response to periodontal therapy in diabetics and smokers. J Periodontol. 1996;67(10 Suppl):1094–102.
19. Grossi SG, Skrepcinski FB, DeCaro T, Robertson DC, Ho AW, Dunford RG, et al. Treatment of periodontal disease in diabetics reduces glycated hemoglobin. J Periodontol. 1997;68:713–9.
20. Stewart JE, Wager KA, Friedlander AH, Zadeh HH. The effect of periodontal treatment on glycemic control in patients with type 2 diabetes mellitus. J Clin Periodontol. 2001;28:306–10.
21. Gerdin EW, Angbratt M, Aronsson K, Eriksson E, Johansson I. Dental caries and body mass index by socio-economic status in Swedish children. Community Dent Oral Epidemiol. 2008;36:459–65.
22. Marshall TA, Eichenberger-Gilmore JM, Broffitt BA, Warren JJ, Levy SM. Dental caries and childhood obesity: roles of diet and socioeconomic status. Community Dent Oral Epidemiol. 2007;35:449–58.
23. de Silva-Sanigorski AM, Waters E, Calache H, Smith M, Gold L, Gussy M, et al. Splash!: a prospective birth cohort study of the impact of environmental, social and family-level influences on child oral health and obesity related risk factors and outcomes. BMC Public Health. 2012;11:505.
24. Malik VS, Hu FB. Sweeteners and risk of obesity and type 2 diabetes: the role of sugar-sweetened beverages. Curr Diab Rep. 2012. [Epub ahead of print].
25. Marshall TA, Levy SM, Broffitt B, Warren JJ, Eichenberger-Gilmore JM, Burns TL, et al. Dental caries and beverage consumption in young children. Pediatrics. 2003;112:e184–91.

Chapter 21
Very Low-Calorie Diets: Saint or Sinner?

Debbie R.J. Cook

There is a new slant on the global health report card. Being overweight is now become more of a global health burden than a lack of nutrition [1]. Obesity is a complex, multifactorial, stigmatizing, and socially ostracizing condition, as well as an important precursor of a number of chronic conditions, including diabetes, hypertension, cardiovascular disease, sleep apnea, cancer, and depression [2]. Any of these individual conditions can be costly in a variety of ways – the financial costs to the health service are far often far outstripped by the human cost to society with poor economical contribution from obese patients with multiple comorbidities who are unable to work and require multiple interventions to keep them healthy [3]. The risk of obesity-related pathology increases as a continuum with rising BMI [4], and obesity also increases the relative risk of developing type two diabetes by 5.3 times in men and 12.7 times in women [5], but more alarmingly there is up to a 40-fold increase in the development of type 2 diabetes in those with a BMI over 35 kg/m^2 [6].

Finding ways to treat obesity therefore becomes an imperative for both society as a whole and individuals. The cornerstones of weight management are always diet and physical

D.R.J. Cook, BSc (Hons), NP, Dip
Center for Health and Human Performance,
76 Harley Street, London W1G 7HH, UK
e-mail: nurseconsultant76@gmail.com, deb.cook@nhs.net

D.W. Haslam et al. (eds.), *Controversies in Obesity*,
DOI 10.1007/978-1-4471-2834-2_21,
© Springer-Verlag London 2014

activity, with behavior change underpinning both. Fad diets should be avoided, as weight is regained immediately the artificial program stops. Unduly restrictive, nutritionally unbalanced diets should not be used because they are ineffective in the long run and can be harmful [7].

In contrast, regimes that reeducate eating habits and that can be permanently maintained have the capacity to induce long-term weight control. Commercial diets provide both individuals and health-care practitioners with a plethora of choice, but the data on the comparative efficacy of these various dietary approaches are lacking. In 2006, a non-blinded randomized trial was performed comparing four popular dietary approaches, and this showed that clinically useful weight loss and fat loss can be achieved using a low-fat, low-carbohydrate, or more conventional low-calorie approach [8]. Since weight-reducing diets come in a variety of guises, they vary not only in their calorific value and composition but also in their effects on disease states and amount of weight loss expected and achieved.

Dietary approaches go in and out of fashion, and patient's choices of nutritional approach are often bizarre and unwieldy, but it is in the practitioner's interest to support the patient to lose weight in the way that suits them best. In a naturalistic study, 54 patients were studied to try to identify personality traits as predictors of success of a multimodal obesity treatment [9]. In this study, there was a variance in weight reduction between 13.6 and 29.8 %, with the higher success rates correlating with those who acted self-expressively in social structures. Very low-calorie diets (VLCDs) and low-carbohydrate approaches are particularly useful then in those patients with busy, active lives; they often respond well to highly prescriptive approaches to nutrition [10].

VLCDs only succeed alongside psychological support, and if the post-diet regime is sufficiently different to the original pre-intervention diet, but can induce degrees of weight loss second only to bariatric surgery, even in the presence of diabetes. In both cases, there is an immediate substantial reduction in the oral consumption of either carbohydrates or substances that can be converted to carbohydrates. VLCDs, however, have the added advantage that the method is non-invasive but still results in a rapid, significant, and often sustainable weight loss; as such they offer an effective and low-cost alternative to bariatric surgery [11]. Modern VLCDs are intended to achieve nutritionally complete balanced meals, without the risk of severe nitrogen and electrolyte imbalances associated with starvation [12].

Origins of VLCDS

VLCDs are not an invention of the twenty-first century. As far back as 1929, a "new" dietary approach was suggested to help to ameliorate the effects of overindulgence in the morbidly obese, when a 400-calorie diet was proposed, reducing the nutritional intake of the obese to 6–8 kcal/kg [13]. This paper was the spearhead to a VLCD diet craze that was eventually a major obesity treatment of the 1980s [14]. The use of hydrolyzed collagen – leftovers from the slaughterhouse floor – as the only protein source, coupled with a lack of added vitamins and balanced electrolytes, resulted in some problems in the early days. In 1973 Dr. Robert Linn was "an amiable, cherubic osteopath" who eventually wrote *The Last Chance Diet* and prescribed VLCDs in the form of a liquid protein-modified fast in plush clinics with "thick carpets and thin nurses," [23] but the diet was thought to lead to an excess of sudden death in young people, based on alteration of QT intervals [24]. The controversy surrounding The Last Chance Diet has lead to a prolonged suspicion of the regimes, although now VLCDS are nutritionally complete, but still attract much negative publicity, not least because of misconceptions surrounding the ketogenic diet. The clinical state of a mild dietary benign ketosis, induced by using VLCDs that contain <50 g of carbohydrate, is often confused with dangerous metabolic ketoacidosis [11].

The VLCDs in use today are standardized by the Codex standardization [15]. VLCDs are defined as diets limiting energy intake to 1.88–3.35 MJ (450–800 kcal) per day, while providing not only daily requirements of trace elements, vitamins, and

TABLE 21.1 Indications and contraindications for VLCDs

Suitable for a VLCD	Caution required	Absolute contraindications
Those with a BMI >30	Age >65 years	Pregnancy/lactation
Those in a structured MDT program for weight loss	Those with a BMI >25 plus one of the comorbidities	Recent angina/MI/stroke
Patients who are in the pathway for bariatric surgery	Those with a BMI <25	Major psychiatric illness
Overweight patients with diabetes, IHD, asthma, IIT in a supervised environment	Children <16/18 years	Severe renal/hepatic disease
	Gout	Malignancy
	Type 1 diabetes	Eating disorder
	Gout/cholelithiasis	Major dysrhythmia

minerals but at least 50 g of high-quality protein and amino acids, and essential fatty acids [16]. This regime is designed to provide rapid weight loss while preserving lean body mass.

Definition of a VLCD

VLCDs are designed to completely replace usual food intake. VLCDs are now considered to be safe and effective, provided they are used under medical supervision and in selected, appropriate individuals [17]. They are not, however, suitable for everyone [18] (Table 21.1).

Diabetes and Other Comorbities

VLCDs have been shown to be the diet most likely to put type 2 diabetes into remission [3]. Several studies have shown a beneficial effect on glycemic control; in an RCT of 75 subjects with diabetes, the use of a VLCD promoted a reduction in fasting glucose, LDL, and total cholesterol levels [19]. A study on 27 obese, type 2 diabetes patients who were given a VLCD in a supervised program found that the VLCD induced considerable weight loss, major improvements in quality of life, and metabolic amelioration [20].

Clinical Use of VLCDS

People on VLCDs for 4–16 weeks report minor side effects such as fatigue, constipation, nausea, and diarrhea, but these conditions usually improve within a few weeks and rarely prevent people from continuing the VLCD. Often patients who have adapted to this way of eating find that their appetite diminishes, and they are far less hungry then they have been before. Gallstones, which frequently develop in obese people (especially women), are even more common during rapid weight loss. The reason for this may be that rapid weight loss appears to decrease the gallbladder's ability to contract bile. But it is unclear whether VLCDs directly cause gallstones or whether the amount of weight loss is responsible for the formation of gallstones [17] or the uncovering of previously existing stones. Temporary hair loss and amenorrhea may occur.

A more serious long-term problem with VLCDs is the rebound effect. Major weight regain (the so-called yo-yo effect) is known to occur [9]. After short-term and rapid weight loss, the uptake of both fatty acids and glucose by adipocytes is increased in order to somehow compensate for the previous weight loss and stress that the cells were under [21]. Many obese patients have great difficulty maintaining weight loss by whatever method over a prolonged period of time and often face gaining much of the weight lost while on a program [9]. A slow, graduated, and phased transition to eating "normal" and healthy meals is advised to ameliorate this tendency.

Finally, reports abounding in the tabloids that calorie restriction can extend life by up to 25 years seem to be greatly exaggerated; very long-term calorie restriction is not generally feasible for human beings [22]. Weight loss using these safe, effective, and evidenced-based programs will help to reduce both the medical and social complications of obesity.

References

1. Hamzelou J. Global health report card. New Sci. 2012;216(2896–2897): 6–7.
2. Kopelman P. Health risks associated with overweight and obesity. Obes Rev. 2007;8:13–7.
3. Slade C. Diabetes-weight management. Ashtead/Surrey: Global Business Media Ltd; 2012.
4. Haslam D. Obesity co-morbidities and the obesity paradox. Pract Diabetes. 2013;30(3):132–5.
5. National Audit Office. Tackling obesity in England; report by the comptroller and auditor general. London: The Stationery Office; 2001.
6. Puhl R, Bownell K. Bias, discrimination and obesity. Obes Res. 2001; 9(12):788–805.
7. NICE. Obesity; Guidance on the prevention, identification, assessment and management of overweight and obesity in adults and children. 2006. Report No.: NICE clinical guideline 43.
8. Truby H, Baic S, deLooy A. Randomised control trial of four commercial weight loss programs in the UK; initial findings from the BBC diet trials. BMJ. 2006;332(7553):1309–14.
9. Lahmann C, Henrich G, Henningsen P, Baessler A, Fischer M, Loew T, et al. The impact of personality traits on the success of a multimodal obesity treatment. Behav Med. 2011;37(4):119–24.
10. Hallam CL, Broom J, Mullins G, Cook D, Haslam D. Comparison of weight loss in patients with type 2 diabetes using a very-low-calorie diet (VLCD) approach. Poster presentation European Congress on Obesity. May 2012.
11. Mullins G, Hallam CL, Broom J. Ketosis, keto-acidosis and very low calorie diets; putting the record straight. Nutr Bull. 2011;36(3):397–402.
12. Saris W. VLCD and sustained weight loss. Obes Res. 2001;9 Suppl 4:295S–301.
13. Evans FaS J. A departure from usual methods in treating obesity. Am J Med Sci. 1929;177:339–48.
14. Bray G. The battle of the bulge; a history of obesity research. Pittsburgh: Dorrance publishing; 2007.
15. DOM UK. Position statement on very low energy diets in the management of obesity. 2007. Available from: http://www.domuk.org/files/very-low-energy-diets.pdf.
16. Team TE. EndNote for iPad getting started guide. New York: Thomson Reuters; 2013.

17. Tsai AG, Wadden TA. The evolution of very-low-calorie diets: an update and meta-analysis. Obesity. 2006;14(8):1283–93.
18. Baker S, Jerums G, Proietto J. Effects and clinical potential of very-low-calorie diets (VLCDs) in type 2 diabetes. Diabetes Res Clin Pract. 2009;85(3):235–42.
19. Yip I, Go V, Desheilds S, Saltsman P, Bellman M, Thames G, et al. Liquid meal replacements and glycaemic control in obese type two diabetes patients. Obes Res. 2001;9(S4):341–7.
20. Snel MaS M. Quality of life in type 2 diabetes mellitus after a very low calorie diet and exercise. Eur J Intern Med. 2012;23:143–9.
21. Eastman Q. Very low calorie diets make adipocytes scream. J Proteome Res. 2009;8(12):5408.
22. Williams EB. Can very low calorie diets increase life expectancy? Br Nutr Found Nutr Bull. 2010;35:152–6.
23. http://www.people.com/people/archive/article/0,,20069895,00.html. Accessed 24 Apr 2013.
24. Isner JM, Sours HE, Paris AL, Ferrans VJ, Roberts WC. Sudden, unexpected death in avid dieters using the liquid-protein-modified-fast diet. Observations in 17 patients and the role of the prolonged QT interval. Circulation. 1979;60:1401–12.

Chapter 22
Obesity and the Mind

David W. Haslam

Obesity is associated with significant increases in lifetime diagnoses of mental health problems including major depression, bipolar disorder, panic disorder, or agoraphobia [1], whereas people with mental illness show a growing incidence of obesity and metabolic syndrome than the general population [2]. Around 45 % of patients seeking help for obesity suffer Axis-1 mental health disorder [3]. However, links between obesity and depression are not clear-cut. In the Swedish Obese Subjects study, severely obese subjects displayed poor mental well-being – depression and anxiety to a similar or greater degree than metastatic malignant melanoma or tetraplegic patients. However, in the same study, suicide rates *increased* postoperatively. Possibly individuals blame their unhappiness on obesity, pin their hopes on reduction, but discover surgery does not improve their unemployment record, finances, or dire family/social circumstances.

Depression

A foremost physician in the eighteenth century was George Cheyne, who suffered from depression at 448 lbs at his peak weight. He described "*Disgust* or *Disrelish* of worldly

D.W. Haslam, MBBS, DGM
Doctor's Surgery, Watton Place Clinic,
60 High Street, Watton at Stone SG143SY, UK
e-mail: dwhaslam@aol.com

D.W. Haslam et al. (eds.), *Controversies in Obesity*,
DOI 10.1007/978-1-4471-2834-2_22,
© Springer-Verlag London 2014

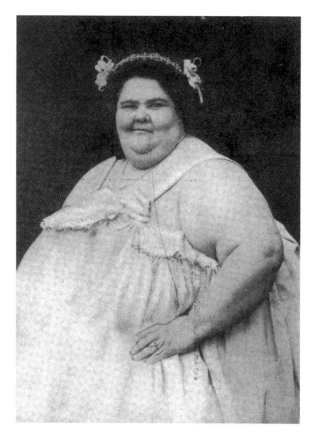

FIGURE 22.1 Jolly Trixie

Amusements and *Creature-Comforts*......tumultuous, overbearing *Hurricanes* in the Mind."

One paper [4] examined links between weight and depression, suicide ideation, and attempts in 40,000 recruits. In women, obesity *increased* diagnoses of major depression by 37 %, but in men obesity *decreased* risk by a similar magnitude. A 10-unit BMI increase increased risk of suicide ideation and attempts in women in the past year by 22 %, while decreasing risks by 26 and 55 %, respectively, in men.

Circus fat people and freak show exhibits often had their name prefixed by "Jolly" (Fig. 22.1). The Texas University asked

"Are Fat People More Jolly?" providing an emphatic "No" [5]. Analyzing BMI, and eight mental health indicators, including overall happiness, relationship satisfaction, and optimism, they discovered "In no case did we observe better mental health among the obese. In sum, the obese were not more jolly."

A Minnesota study [6] assessed psychological effects of overeating in 5,000 students; 17 % of girls and 8 % of boys reported what they considered as binge eating, but only 3 % of girls and 1 % of boys actually met binge eating disorder criteria. Twenty-nine percent of girls who reported overeating, and 28 % of boys, said they had tried to kill themselves, compared to only 10 % of the rest. A National Obesity Forum poll revealed that over half of overweight people lack self-confidence, especially young women, notably when swimming, exercising, holidaying, or in pubs. Forty-one percent felt judged more because of their weight than any other characteristic; 25 % had been insulted by children. Conversely, a third of normal-weight individuals confess to treating overweight people differently; 25 % believe that overweight people simply lack control. Stunkard quotes a patient describing herself: "a great mass of gray-green, amorphous material. Then at times I feel like a sloth. And just now, when I got up on the examining table, I felt like an elephant."

Schizophrenic individuals have life expectancy ~20 years less than the general population, with high obesity rates and CVD mortality. In one study, obese schizophrenia patients had a mean vascular age 14.1 years older than their actual age, whereas obese NHANES participants had only a 6.7-year difference. The probability of experiencing a CVD event within 10 years was 10.7 % for obese schizophrenia patients and 8.5 % for obese NHANES participants [7].

Binge Eating Disorder

Binge eating disorder (BED) is common, misunderstood, poorly recognized, and badly treated, with devastating consequences. The Diagnostic and Statistical Manual of Mental Disorders (DSM) [8] is the broadly accepted manual for mental illness classification, published by the American Psychiatric Association;

DSM-5 is the latest incarnation. Allen Frances was chair of the DSM-IV Task Force and describes aspects of DSM-5 as "breathtakingly wrong-headed [exceeding] even my most pessimistic expectations about DSM-5's lack of competence and credibility" [9]. The labelling of grief as major depression and the increased emphasis of female sexual dysfunction as a pharmaceutical target are two controversial aspects. However, in obesity-related eating disorders, changes could be an improvement. The category EDNOS (Eating Disordered Not Otherwise Specified) has shrunk; anorexia no longer requires amenorrhea as a criterion, allowing males to be diagnosed; and BED has finally been recognized in its own right. The latter change will, at last, facilitate insurance claims and improve access to cognitive therapy and other techniques, stopping patients being turned away from clinics because "obesity is not an eating disorder." BED represents a public health problem at least equal to bulimia nervosa, but its management has been compromised by lack of recognition; fewer than half of patients ever receive treatment [10]. Critics say inclusion is medicalizing a style of eating in normal individuals, others that BED signifies an underlying disorder which will now go undetected [11].

Like obesity, BED is generally put down by the public to lack of self-discipline [12], whereas loss of control is considered a hallmark symptom [13]. Abnormal neural pathways [14] and genetic predisposition [15] have been put forward as causes, and there are links with depression, personality disorders, obsessive-compulsive disorders [16], and social anxiety [17]. BED sufferers display features of bulimia nervosa, without compensatory weight-loss-inducing features: purging or abnormal exercise regimes. It was initially recognized, but largely ignored, in the 1950s; criteria are loss of control of eating plus three of the following:

• Eating much more rapidly than normal
• Eating until uncomfortably full
• Eating large amounts when not physically hungry
• Eating alone because of embarrassment of volume of consumption
• Feeling disgusted, depressed, or very guilty afterward

Studies suggest that 2.5 % of adult women and 1.1 % of men suffer from BED, of whom most but not all are obese [18]. The prevalence among patients attending obesity clinics is 20–30 %, emphasizing the importance of prompt recognition. The treatment of choice is cognitive behavioral therapy (CBT) [19], without which developing normal patterns and regaining control of eating are unlikely to succeed.

Albert Stunkard quoted the patient who first made him consider the existence of BED, a man named Hyman Cohen, "… 'everything seemed to go blank. I just said 'what the Hell' and started eating.' He started with cake, pieces of pie, and cookies, then set out on a furtive round of the local restaurants, then went to a delicatessen, bought another $20 of food 'until my gut ached. I'll drink beer, maybe six or eight bottles to keep me going, then I'll want more food. I don't feel in control any more. I feel like Hell. I should be punished for the shameful act I've performed.'"

Secretive food concocting – combining bizarre foods, such as mashed potatoes and Oreo cookies, or frozen vegetables with mayonnaise – can be a feature of BED [20]. "While they are food concocting and binge eating they report being excited, in a frenzy, and high, but afterwards they feel awful about themselves" [21].

Night Eating Syndrome

Night eating syndrome (NES), like BED, was described by Stunkard in the 1950s and is associated with psychological and emotional factors, sufferers frequently being moody, tense, anxious, nervous, and depressed. There are changes in the circadian rhythm and disruption of the hypothalamo-pituitary axis.

Symptoms and criteria are as follows [22]:

- Daily eating pattern demonstrates significantly increased intake in the evening and/or night time, as manifested by one or both of the following:

  - ≥25 % of food intake consumed after the evening meal.
  - At least two episodes of nocturnal eating per week.

- Awareness and recall of evening and nocturnal episodes are present.
- The clinical picture is characterized by at least three of the following:
  - Lack of desire to eat in the morning and/or breakfast is omitted on ≥4 mornings per week.
  - Strong urge to eat between dinner and sleep onset and/or during the night.
  - Belief that one must eat to initiate or return to sleep.
  - Sleep onset and/or sleep maintenance insomnia is present >4 nights per week.
  - Mood frequently depressed and/or mood worsens in the evening.
- Association with significant distress and/or impairment in functioning.
- The disordered eating pattern has been maintained for at least 3 months.
- The disorder is not secondary to substance abuse or dependence, medical disorder, medication, or another psychiatric disorder.

Population prevalence is ~1–2 %, rising to 25 % of obese patients in some studies [23]. It is associated with obstructive sleep apnea and restless legs syndrome, but links with nocturnal sleep-related eating disorder (NS-RED) are unclear. NS-RED [24] is a sleep disorder rather than an eating disorder characterized by eating during sleep – like sleep walking – without recollection, whereas NES patients recall nocturnal eating. A study of NES [25] emphasized lack of hunger prior to episodes of night eating, "automaticity" of behavior during waking intervals, and varying levels of consciousness during eating. Many sufferers eat fast and carelessly, 30 % having injured themselves. Treatment has been attempted by behavioral therapy, phototherapy, behavioral weight-loss treatment, and cognitive behavioral therapy to regain normal eating patterns [26]. Circadian rhythms are reinforced by appropriate exercise during the day, normal regular mealtimes, and daily routines. Escitalopram has been used successfully [27].

Food Addiction

The existence of food addiction is contentious. Robert Lustig's "Fat Chance" [28] famously reviews the science around sugar, updating John Yudkin's seminal and brave work [29], and is dedicated to "those of you who eat food. The rest of you are off the hook." His description of addictiveness of sugar is compelling [30], explaining the biochemical negative feedback induced by leptin, which should prevent caloric excess and its disruption. Leptin stimulates hypothalamic melanocortin systems, decreasing caloric intake and increasing energy expenditure. Also, in the ventral tegmental area and nucleus accumbens (VTA-NA), leptin reduces dopamine neurotransmission, attenuating "reward." When leptin falls, the opposite happens – increased food intake with increased reward. In obesity, leptin resistance occurs – linked with hypertriglyceridemia, insulin resistance, and hyperinsulinemia – diminishing its effects, disrupting the body's fine-tuning in controlling weight, and providing the link with obesity. Sugar, as the prime suspect, also has a direct effect on the VTA-NA, which in animal experiments has shown to induce bingeing, withdrawal, craving, and cross-sensitization with other drugs. Obesity and drug addiction exhibit similar effects on dopamine.

However, a recent paper concluded that food addiction's significance is unknown and needs validating in prospective studies [31]. Unsurprisingly, chocolate has been studied for addictiveness: many attractive theories surrounding caffeine, theobromine, phenylethylamine, and tyramine are proposed, but it is possible that chocolate craving is merely for enjoyable sensory experience and nothing to do with addiction. It has been suggested that endogenous opioids are to blame, while another recent paper [32] adds to literature regarding dopamine: subjects could see and smell their favorite food, and even without even tasting, dopamine levels increased, the conclusion being that we eat for more than just simple hunger.

Depraved Appetites

In 1771 Goldschmidt of Weimar met a traveler in the woods, accused him of cow frightening, killed him with a stick, dragged the body to the bushes, cut it up, took it home in pieces, and ate it. He developed a taste for human meat and was eventually caught eating an abducted child. Another deranged cannibal, Menesclou, was caught with a missing child's forearm in his pocket and in his stove the child's head and entrails; in his defense he claimed the situation was "an accident." The famous French glutton Tarrare was accused of eating a 14-month-old child and, perhaps unsurprisingly, died of diarrhea. The "Great Eater of Kent" was the name given to Nicholas Wood, the subject of John Taylor's 1630 work "the admirable teeth and stomach exploits of Nicholas Wood, of Harrisom in the county of Kent, His excessive manner of Eating without manners in strange and true manner described." Wood's gluttonous feats are recorded in detail by the incredulous writer: "Once at Sir Warham Saint Ledger's house, he shewed himself so valiant of teeth and stomach, that he ate as much as would well have served and sufficed thirty men, so that his belly was like to turn bankrupt and break, but that the serving-men turned him to the fire, and anointed his paunch with grease and butter, to make it stretch and hold." Wood was known as a "Tugmutton" for being one of a small group of people to have eaten a whole sheep, raw at a single sitting, except for skin, wool, horns, and bones.

References

1. Simon GE, Von Korff M, Saunders K, Miglioretti DL, Crane PK, van Belle G, Kessler RC. Association between obesity and psychiatric disorders in the US adult population. Arch Gen Psychiatry. 2006;63: 824–30.
2. Stanley SH, Laugharne JD. Obesity, cardiovascular disease and type 2 diabetes in people with a mental illness: a need for primary health care. Aust J Prim Health. 2012;18(3):258–64.

3. Carpiniello B, Pinna F, Velluzzi F, Loviselli A. Mental disorders in patients with metabolic syndrome. The key role of central obesity. Eat Weight Disord. 2012;17(4):e259–66.

4. Carpenter KM, Hasin DS, Allison DB, Faith MS. Relationships between obesity and DSM-IV major depressive disorder, suicide ideation, and suicide attempts: results from a general population study. Am J Public Health. 2000;90:251–71.

5. Roberts R, Strawbridge W, Deleger S, Kaplan G. Are the fat more jolly? Ann Behav Med. 2002;24(3):169–80.

6. Ackard D, Neumark-Sztainer D, Story M, Perry C. Overeating among adolescents: prevalence and associations with weight-related characteristics and psychological health. Pediatrics. 2003;111:67–74.

7. Ratliff JC, Palmese LB, Reutenauer EL, Srihari VH, Tek C. Obese schizophrenia spectrum patients have significantly higher 10-year general cardiovascular risk and vascular ages than obese individuals without severe mental illness. Psychosomatics. 2013;54(1):67–73.

8. http://www.dsm5.org/Pages/Default.aspx.

9. Frances AJ. DSM5 in distress. Psychology today. 2013. http://www.psychologytoday.com/blog/dsm5-in-distress/201301/bad-news-dsm-5-refuses-correct-somatic-symptom-disorder. Accessed 8 Apr 2013.

10. Kessler RC, Berglund PA, Chiu WT, Deitz AC, Hudson JI, Shahly V, et al. The prevalence and correlates of binge eating disorder in the World Health Organization World Mental Health Surveys. Biol Psychiatry. 2013;73(9):904–14. pii: S0006-3223(12)01028-1.

11. http://ct.counseling.org/2012/12/binge-eating-disorder-to-be-recognized-in-the-dsm-v/. Accessed 15 Apr 2013.

12. Ebneter DS, Latner JD. Stigmatizing attitudes differ across mental health disorders: a comparison of stigma across eating disorders, obesity, and major depressive disorder. J Nerv Ment Dis. 2013;201(4): 281–5.

13. Vannucci A, Theim KR, Kass AE, Trockel M, Genkin B, Rizk M, et al. What constitutes clinically significant binge eating? Association between binge features and clinical validators in college-age women. Int J Eat Disord. 2013;46(3):226–32.

14. Balodis IM, Molina ND, Kober H, Worhunsky PD, White MA, Rajita Sinha, et al. Divergent neural substrates of inhibitory control in binge eating disorder relative to other manifestations of obesity. Obesity (Silver Spring). 2013;21(2):367–77.

15. Trace SE, Baker JH, Peñas-Lledó E, Bulik CM. The genetics of eating disorders. Annu Rev Clin Psychol. 2013;9:589–620.

16. Pollack LO, Forbush KT. Why do eating disorders and obsessive-compulsive disorder co-occur? Eat Behav. 2013;14(2):211–5.

17. Ostrovsky NW, Swencionis C, Wylie-Rosett J, Isasi CR. Social anxiety and disordered overeating: an association among overweight and obese individuals. Eat Behav. 2013;14(2):145–8.

18. Spitzer RL, Yanovski S, Wadden T, Wing R, Marcus MD, Stunkard A, et al. Binge eating disorder: its further validation in a multisite study. Int J Eat Disord. 1993;13(2):137–53.

19. Spielmans GI, Benish SG, Marin C, Bowman WM, Menster M, Wheeler AJ. Specificity of psychological treatments for bulimia nervosa and binge eating disorder? A meta-analysis of direct comparisons. Clin Psychol Rev. 2013;33(3):460–9.

20. Boggiano MM, Turan B, Maldonado CR, Oswald KD, Shuman ES. Secretive food concocting in binge eating: test of a famine hypothesis. Int J Eat Disord. 2013;46(3):212–25.

21. http://www.sciencedaily.com/releases/2013/01/130103130754.htm.

22. Allison KC, Lundgren JD, O'Reardon JP, Geliebter A, Gluck ME, Vinai P, et al. Proposed diagnostic criteria for night eating syndrome. Int J Eat Disord. 2010;43:241–7.

23. Cleator J, Abbott J, Judd P, Sutton C, Wilding JPH. Night eating syndrome: implications for severe obesity. Nutr Diabetes. 2012;2(9):e44.

24. Vetrugno R, Manconi M, Ferini-Strambi L, Provini F, Plazzi G, Montagna P. Nocturnal eating: sleep-related eating disorder or night eating syndrome? A videopolysomnographic study. Sleep. 2006;29(7):949–54.

25. Schenck CH, Mahowald MW. Review of nocturnal sleep-related eating disorders. Eat Disord. 1994;15(4):343–56.

26. Berner LA, Allison KC. Behavioral management of night eating disorders. Psychol Res Behav Manag. 2013;6:1–8. Epub 2013 Mar 28.

27. Allison KC, Studt SK, Berkowitz RI, Hesson LA, Moore RH, Dubroff JG, et al. An open-label efficacy trial of escitalopram for night eating syndrome. Eat Behav. 2013;14(2):199–203. Epub 2013 Mar 5.

28. Lustig R. Fat chance. The bitter truth about sugar. New York: Hudson Street Press; 2012.

29. Yudkin J. Pure, white and deadly. New York: Penguin; 1972.

30. Avena NM, Rada P, Hoebel BG. Evidence for sugar addiction: behavioural and neurochemical effects of intermittent. Excessive sugar intake. Neurosci Biobehav Rev. 2008;32:20–39.

31. Eichen DM, Lent MR, Goldbacher E, Foster GD. Exploration of "food addiction" in overweight and obese treatment-seeking adults. Appetite. 2013;67:22–4. pii: S0195-6663(13)00098-6.

32. Salamone JD, Correa M. Dopamine and food addiction: lexicon badly needed. Biol Psychiatry. 2013;73(9):e15–24. pii: S0006-3223(12)00853-0.

Chapter 23
Adipose Tissue Expansion for Improving Glycemic Control

Nikhil V. Dhurandhar

Background

Obesity is linked with metabolic abnormalities [1, 2], which improve upon weight loss [3–5]. Lifestyle modification and anti-obesity drugs in appropriately selected cases are the best and the only major nonsurgical obesity treatment options available to clinicians. These available obesity-management approaches work well for some responders but do not achieve adequate and lasting benefits for the majority. It is hard to continue promoting the use of weight loss approaches to improve metabolic health, when nonresponders or poor responders often outnumber the responders. A potentially alternative approach is to develop approaches that improve the comorbidities of obesity without a reduction in adiposity. While this approach may not be appropriate for improving every obesity-related comorbidity, the point is illustrated below, by using glycemic control as an example.

Although obesity reduction is justifiably considered integral to diabetes prevention or treatment, due to poor success

N.V. Dhurandhar, PhD
Infections and Obesity Lab,
Pennington Biomedical Research Center,
Louisiana State University System, 6400 Perkins Road,
Baton Rouge, LA 70808, USA
e-mail: nikhil.dhurandhar@pbrc.edu

D.W. Haslam et al. (eds.), *Controversies in Obesity*,   185
DOI 10.1007/978-1-4471-2834-2_23,
© Springer-Verlag London 2014

of weight loss and maintenance strategies, the benefits of weight loss mainly remain theoretical. Besides, not all obese individuals develop diabetes, and obesity reduction may not necessarily benefit universally [6]. A closer examination reveals that it is not obesity per se, but more specific factors, such as excessive hepatic fat accumulation or circulating excess lipids, which may play a primary role in impaired glycemic control. Ectopic deposition of fat, particularly in liver, is associated with adverse metabolic health and glycemic control [7], independent of total body fat [8, 9]. It has been argued that it is the circulating fat and not the "stored fat" that is a determinant of glycemic control [10]. This implies that fat accumulation is a metabolically "inert" event, until it exceeds the storage capacity of adipose tissue and other organs and "spills over" in circulation. Possibly, it is the lipotoxicity that ensues when the lipid storage capacity of adipose tissue and organs such as liver is exceeded and leads to a derangement in mitochondrial function, inflammatory process, or endoplasmic reticular or oxidative stress, which in turn may contribute to insulin resistance [10]. Therefore, reducing ectopic fat deposition or the circulating fat appears to be a better target for preventing and treating diabetes. Reducing obesity is but one approach to achieve this [11].

Another approach to reduce circulating or ectopic fat may be to increase lipid storage capacity of the adipose tissue. In fact, an impaired ability of adipose tissue expansion contributes to insulin resistance and other metabolic abnormalities [12, 13]. Preadipocytes of diabetic individuals have impaired ability for adipogenic differentiation [14]. Conversely, an increase in adipogenesis is a key enhancer of glycemic control [15]. Thiazolidinedione (TZD) class of drugs, which are agonists of peroxisome proliferator-activated receptor gamma (PPARγ), offers perhaps the most notable example of enhanced adipogenesis coupled with antidiabetic effects [16]. As PPARγ is a master regulator of adipogenesis, the TZDs upregulate adipogenesis, increase adiposity, yet improve glycemic control [17].

The contribution of adipogenesis to improving glycemic control is nicely documented in animal models. Several transgenic animal models show that adipose tissue expansion under specific circumstances is associated with better glycemic profile of animals. Transgenic mice that overexpress glucose transporter Glut4 in adipose tissue [18] show significantly greater fat-cell number, threefold greater lipid accumulation, greater body weight, yet a significantly better glycemic control. Additional animal models showed that the expansion of adipose tissue achieved by overexpression of adipocytokines, adiponectin, or tartrate-resistant acid phosphatase (TRAP) significantly increases adiposity yet shows a remarkable improvement in glycemic control [19, 20]. Collagen VI offers a casing for adipose tissue and limits its uncontrolled expansion. A knockdown of collagen VI allows the expansion of adipose tissue, and yet the mice have a better glycemic control [21]. Similarly, Ad36, a human adenovirus, increases adiposity in experimentally infected animals on the one hand and yet improves glycemic control in these animals [22, 23]. In humans, natural infection of Ad36 is associated with obesity [24] and better glycemic control [22] (see also Chap. 7).

Despite their greater whole body adiposity, these animal models show significantly lower hepatic lipid content, lower plasma triglycerides, and/or quicker lipid clearance from circulation, compared to their respective controls [19, 21, 22, 25], which probably contributes to their better glycemic profile. Humans who were naturally infected with Ad36 also showed lower hepatic lipid content [26] and better glycemic control [22]. The precise underlying mechanisms that contribute to enhanced glycemic control may vary by the model of adipogenesis. However, a common underlying explanation may be that adipogenesis and adipose tissue expansion sequester circulating fat, a phenomenon known as "lipid steal," which prevents fat from getting stored ectopically in skeletal muscle, liver, or other organs and thus improves glycemic control [27].

These examples indicate that it is possible to improve glycemic control, without reducing adiposity, and in certain situations, even increasing adipogenesis/adiposity may help. Therefore, while sound in theory, obesity reduction does not appear to be a practical and widely applicable solution for improving diabetes. In contrast, expansion of adipose tissue offers a conceptually different approach to reduce ectopic fat deposition and circulating lipids for improving glycemic control. Admittedly, iatrogenic weight gain to improve diabetes may be socially and cosmetically undesirable and inappropriate for some other obesity-associated comorbidities. Therefore, it is less practical to promote adipogenesis as a measure to improve glycemic control. Instead, this approach provides templates and targets for developing weight loss-independent antidiabetic strategies. It is expected that future research could creatively uncouple the adipogenic and anti-glycemic effects as illustrated below.

For instance, adenovirus Ad36 or the TZDs upregulate PPARγ and influence adipogenesis and glycemic control. However, Ad36 can increase cellular glucose uptake even in complete absence of PPARγ [28]. Also, limiting the activation of PPARγ specifically to adipocytes, insulin sensitivity can be improved without increasing adipogenesis [29]. Moreover, efforts to either completely or partially bypass PPARγ activation or its downstream signaling are under investigation for promoting glucose uptake [28, 30, 31]. Another approach is to focus on adiponectin, a target gene of PPARγ and a key insulin sensitizer. The currently known main strategies to increase adiponectin include weight loss or PPARγ activation via the TZDs [32, 33]. However, it may be possible to enhance adiponectin without weight loss or PPARγ activation [28, 34]. The antidiabetic action of the TZDs appears to be due to the ability to block PPARγ phosphorylation, which enhances adiponectin [34]. The blockade of PPARγ phosphorylation and upregulation of adiponectin can also be achieved by other compounds with minimal PPARγ activation and adipogenic potential [34].

In summary, it is intuitive to attempt weight loss to alleviate obesity-associated metabolic abnormalities, such as diabetes. However, to achieve and sustain meaningful weight loss is hard for a majority of the free-living population. Somewhat paradoxically, even an expansion of adipose tissue can improve glycemic control under specific circumstances. This phenomenon provides a template to be creatively exploited for improving obesity-associated metabolic abnormalities independent of weight loss.

Acknowledgment   Dr. Dhurandhar holds the following US patents: patent number 6,127,113 (Viral obesity methods and compositions), patent number 6,664,050 (Viral obesity methods and compositions), patent number US 8,008,436B2, dated August 30, 2011 (Adenovirus 36 E4orf1 gene and protein and their uses), provisional patent filed (Adenovirus Ad36 E4orf1 protein for prevention and treatment of non-alcoholic fatty liver disease, July 2010), and provisional patent filed (Enhanced glycemic control using Ad36E4orf1 and AKT1 Inhibitor, January 2012).

References

1. BerringtondeGonzalez A, Hartge P, Cerhan JR, Flint AJ, Hannan L, et al. Body-mass index and mortality among 1.46 million white adults. N Engl J Med. 2010;363:2211–9.
2. Wormser D, Kaptoge S, Di Angelantonio E, Wood AM, Pennells L, Thompson A, et al. Separate and combined associations of body-mass index and abdominal adiposity with cardiovascular disease: collaborative analysis of 58 prospective studies. Lancet. 2011;377: 1085–95.
3. Unick JL, Beavers D, Jakicic JM, Kitabchi AE, Knowler WC, Wadden TA, et al. Effectiveness of lifestyle interventions for individuals with severe obesity and type 2 diabetes: results from the look AHEAD trial. Diabetes Care. 2011;34:2152–7.
4. Wing RR. Long-term effects of a lifestyle intervention on weight and cardiovascular risk factors in individuals with type 2 diabetes mellitus: four-year results of the look AHEAD trial. Arch Intern Med. 2010;170:1566–75.
5. Hamman RF, Wing RR, Edelstein SL, Lachin JM, Bray GA, Delahanty L, et al. Effect of weight loss with lifestyle intervention on risk of diabetes. Diabetes Care. 2006;29:2102–7.
6. Eckel RH, Kahn SE, Ferrannini E, Goldfine AB, Nathan DM, Schwartz MW, et al. Obesity and type 2 diabetes: what can be unified and what needs to be individualized? Diabetes Care. 2011;34: 1424–30.
7. Kotronen A, Yki-Jarvinen H, Sevastianova K, Bergholm R, Hakkarainen A, Pietilainen KH, et al. Comparison of the relative contributions of intra-abdominal and liver fat to components of the metabolic syndrome. Obesity. 2011;19:23–8.
8. Fabbrini E, Magkos F, Mohammed BS, Pietka T, Abumrad NA, Patterson BW, et al. Intrahepatic fat, not visceral fat, is linked with metabolic complications of obesity. Proc Natl Acad Sci U S A. 2009; 106:15430–5.
9. Magkos F, Fabbrini E, Mohammed BS, Patterson BW, Klein S. Increased whole-body adiposity without a concomitant increase in liver fat is not associated with augmented metabolic dysfunction. Obesity (Silver Spring). 2010;18(8):1510–5.

10. Sorensen TI. Obesity defined as excess storage of inert triglycerides–do we need a paradigm shift? Obes Facts. 2011;4:91–4.

11. Vitola BE, Deivanayagam S, Stein RI, Mohammed BS, Magkos F, Kirk EP, Klein S. Weight loss reduces liver fat and improves hepatic and skeletal muscle insulin sensitivity in obese adolescents. Obesity (Silver Spring). 2009;17:1744–8.

12. Arner P, Arner E, Hammarstedt A, Smith U. Genetic predisposition for type 2 diabetes, but not for overweight/obesity, is associated with a restricted adipogenesis. PLoS One. 2011;6:e18284.

13. Garg A. Lipodystrophies. Am J Med. 2000;108:143–52.

14. van Tienen FH, van der Kallen CJ, Lindsey PJ, Wanders RJ, van Greevenbroek MM, Smeets HJ. Preadipocytes of type 2 diabetes subjects display an intrinsic gene expression profile of decreased differentiation capacity. Int J Obes. 2011;35:1154–64.

15. Tan CY, Vidal-Puig A. Adipose tissue expandability: the metabolic problems of obesity may arise from the inability to become more obese. Biochem Soc Trans. 2008;36:935–40.

16. Staels B, Fruchart JC. Therapeutic roles of peroxisome proliferator-activated receptor agonists. Diabetes. 2005;54:2460–70.

17. Larsen TM, Toubro S, Astrup A. PPARgamma agonists in the treatment of type II diabetes: is increased fatness commensurate with long-term efficacy? Int J Obes Relat Metab Disord. 2003;27:147–61.

18. Shepherd PR, Gnudi L, Tozzo E, Yang H, Leach F, Kahn BB. Adipose cell hyperplasia and enhanced glucose disposal in transgenic mice overexpressing GLUT4 selectively in adipose tissue. J Biol Chem. 1993;268:22243–6.

19. Kim JY, van de Wall E, Laplante M, Azzara A, Trujillo ME, Hofmann SM, et al. Obesity-associated improvements in metabolic profile through expansion of adipose tissue. J Clin Invest. 2007;117:2621–37.

20. Lang P, van Harmelen V, Ryden M, Kaaman M, Parini P, Carneheim C, et al. Monomeric tartrate resistant acid phosphatase induces insulin sensitive obesity. PLoS One. 2008;3:e1713.

21. Khan T, Muise ES, Iyengar P, Wang ZV, Chandalia M, Abate N, et al. Metabolic dysregulation and adipose tissue fibrosis: role of collagen VI. Mol Cell Biol. 2009;29:1575–91.

22. Krishnapuram R, Dhurandhar EJ, Dubuisson O, Kirk-Ballard H, Bajpeyi S, Butte N, et al. Template to improve glycemic control without reducing adiposity or dietary fat. Am J Physiol Endocrinol Metab. 2011;300:E779–89.

23. Pasarica M, Shin AC, Yu M, Ou Yang HM, Rathod M, Jen KL, et al. Human adenovirus 36 induces adiposity, increases insulin sensitivity, and alters hypothalamic monoamines in rats. Obesity (Silver Spring). 2006;14:1905–13.

24. Dhurandhar NV. A framework for identification of infections that contribute to human obesity. Lancet Infect Dis. 2011;11:963–9.

25. Johmura Y, Watanabe K, Kishimoto K, Ueda T, Shimada S, Osada S, et al. Fad24 causes hyperplasia in adipose tissue and improves glucose metabolism. Biol Pharm Bull. 2009;32:1656–64.

26. Trovato GM, Martines GF, Garozzo A, Tonzuso A, Timpanaro R, Pirri C, et al. Ad36 adipogenic adenovirus in human non-alcoholic fatty liver disease. Liver Int. 2010;30:184–90.

27. Ye JM, Dzamko N, Cleasby ME, Hegarty BD, Furler SM, Cooney GJ, et al. Direct demonstration of lipid sequestration as a mechanism by which rosiglitazone prevents fatty-acid-induced insulin resistance in the rat: comparison with metformin. Diabetologia. 2004;47:1306–13.

28. Dubuisson O, Dhurandhar EJ, Krishnapuram R, Kirk-Ballard H, Gupta AK, Hegde V, et al. PPAR{gamma}-independent increase in glucose uptake and adiponectin abundance in fat cells. Endocrinology. 2011;152(10):3648–60.

29. Sugii S, Olson P, Sears DD, Saberi M, Atkins AR, Barish GD, et al. PPARgamma activation in adipocytes is sufficient for systemic insulin sensitization. Proc Natl Acad Sci U S A. 2009;106:22504–9.

30. Knouff C, Auwerx J. Peroxisome proliferator-activated receptor-gamma calls for activation in moderation: lessons from genetics and pharmacology. Endocr Rev. 2004;25:899–918.

31. Mukherjee R, Hoener PA, Jow L, Bilakovics J, Klausing K, Mais DE, et al. A selective peroxisome proliferator-activated receptor-gamma (PPAR-gamma) modulator blocks adipocyte differentiation but stimulates glucose uptake in 3T3-L1 adipocytes. Mol Endocrinol. 2000;14:1425–33.

32. Boden G, Cheung P, Mozzoli M, Fried SK. Effect of thiazolidinediones on glucose and fatty acid metabolism in patients with type 2 diabetes. Metabolism. 2003;52:753–9.

33. Engl J, Bobbert T, Ciardi C, Laimer M, Tatarczyk T, Kaser S, et al. Effects of pronounced weight loss on adiponectin oligomer composition and metabolic parameters. Obesity (Silver Spring). 2007;15:1172–8.

34. Choi JH, Banks AS, Estall JL, Kajimura S, Bostrom P, Laznik D, et al. Anti-diabetic drugs inhibit obesity-linked phosphorylation of PPARgamma by Cdk5. Nature. 2010;466:451–6.

Chapter 24
Should Hip and Knee Arthroplasty Be Restricted in the Obese?

Tim S. Waters

The risk of developing degenerative joint disease is substantially increased in obese patients [1, 2]. As the obese population grows, it is likely that more patients will present for consideration of joint replacement surgery.

In the UK, health authorities have imposed restrictions on joint replacement surgery in patients with an elevated body mass index (BMI), typically above 30–35 [3, 4] – the premise being to avoid surgical complications and promote a healthier lifestyle.

Are the Risks and Outcomes of Joint Replacement in This Group Significant Enough to Warrant Restriction?

No surgery is risk-free, and the specific risks of total hip and knee replacement include wound problems, infection, deep vein thrombosis (DVT), pulmonary embolism (PE), and failure of the implants. Hence, joint replacement surgery is generally

T.S. Waters, MBBS, MRCS, FRCS (Orth)
The Hip and Knee Unit, West Hertfordshire
Hospitals NHS Trust, Vicarage Road, Watford,
Hertfordshire WD18 0HB, UK
e-mail: mail@timwaters.com

D.W. Haslam et al. (eds.), *Controversies in Obesity*, 193
DOI 10.1007/978-1-4471-2834-2_24,
© Springer-Verlag London 2014

only performed when all conservative measures have failed. The results of hip and knee arthroplasty are multifactorial: severity of arthropathy, age, gender, ethnicity, socioeconomic status, and other comorbidities correlate better with outcome rather than obesity [5–9].

There is little substantial evidence relating obesity to poor outcome in hip replacement surgery. In 1,421 hip replacements followed up to 9 years, there was no difference in outcome scores, complications, or radiographic appearances. There was also no difference in the prevalence of PE, infection, dislocation, or revision [10]. In 3,290 hip replacements stratified according to BMI, there was an overall greater improvement in outcome scores in overweight patients [11].

Some studies suggest increased perioperative problems such as DVT, PE, and wound problems with obese patients undergoing knee replacement [9, 12, 13]. However, the majority of publications suggest that there is no significant difference in the moderately obese [3, 4, 14–16]. Out of 9,735 knee prostheses, there were no significantly different rates of survival or perioperative complications in 3,031 obese subjects compared with normal-weight subjects, at a minimum of 5 years [17]. In 370 consecutive knee replacements, there was no difference in outcome/complication rates looking at BMI, gender, and absolute weight at 5 years [18].

In the morbidly obese (BMI >40), a higher rate of complications, particularly wound infection, has been noted [8, 19]. Surgery is also technically demanding in these cases, with an increased operating time and larger incisions. Most studies have demonstrated high patient satisfaction, and while weight loss is desirable, it should not necessarily be a barrier to surgery [9–11, 19–30].

Recovery from hip and knee replacement surgery has improved dramatically over the last few years with the introduction of enhanced recovery programs. Patient education, combined with early mobilization and a variety of anesthetic and surgical techniques, has started to facilitate the early discharge of patients while minimizing complications [31]. The author's experience of 1,000 patients in an enhanced recovery pathway (including 454 obese and 34 morbidly obese cases) showed no difference in length of stay, wound complications,

DVT, or blood transfusion requirements [32]. In another study, no significant influence of individual BMI was observed in length of stay or outcome at either 10 days or 3 months after surgery [33]. Others have demonstrated no increase in hospital resources [34].

Hip and knee replacement surgery have been shown to be a cost-effective way of dramatically improving quality of life, whatever the BMI of the patient [35, 36]. A "poorer" outcome (i.e., not walking as far or functioning quite as well as their nonobese counterparts) is not the same as a "poor outcome." While obese patients may have lower outcome scores, their quality of life still improves significantly. Outcome scores tend to be lower pre- and postoperatively in obese patients; however, the change in scores, satisfaction, and revision rates is similar [30, 37]. In fact, quality-of-life outcomes have been shown to be greater in the obese even if the overall score is lower [21, 23]. In one study of both hip and knee replacement surgery, quality-of-life measures improved more for obese patients than for patients with ideal body weight [38].

Hip and knee prostheses do not appear to wear out more quickly in the overweight, possibly due to sedentary activity [16, 37, 39, 40]. In fact, a higher prevalence of radiological evidence of wear has been observed in normal-weight patients [41, 42].

Does Weight Loss Reverse the Need for Joint Replacement Surgery?

Although weight loss may improve function, it has little impact on pain [43]. Studies do show a benefit from weight loss on symptoms of early degenerative change [44–46]. However, no studies have ever been performed to see if patients whose disease is severe enough to require joint replacement surgery can avoid an operation through weight loss. Degenerative joint disease is irreversible, and it is unlikely that patients with pain from bone-on-bone arthritis, with deformation of the joint, would find their symptoms altered greatly, particularly in the hip.

Patients often claim that painful joints limit exercise and weight loss. While it may indeed be the case that the pain prevents meaningful exercise, it does not prevent calorie control. Interestingly, the majority of patients tend not to lose weight after hip [47] or knee replacement surgery [48]. This in itself is not a reason to withhold surgery, but rather, there is a role for a weight loss program after surgery is performed [49]. There may be a role for preoperative bariatric surgery for selected patients [39, 50].

Conclusion

Hip and knee replacements are successful, quality-of-life changing operations that have revolutionized the treatment of degenerative joint disease. Modern techniques allow rapid return to pain-free function. Weight loss in the obese is to be encouraged for a myriad of health-related benefits. Patients should certainly be counselled regarding the relative risks of surgery, particularly the morbidly obese undergoing knee replacement. However, the evidence suggests that withholding a pain-relieving operation in cases where conservative treatments have failed is unjustified and, in the author's opinion, unethical.

References

1. Ackerman IN, Osborne RH. Obesity and increased burden of hip and knee joint disease in Australia: results from a national survey. BMC Musculoskelet Disord. 2012;13(1):254.
2. Bourne R, Mukhi S, Zhu N, Keresteci M, Marin M. Role of obesity on the risk for total hip or knee arthroplasty. Clin Orthop Relat Res. 2007;465:185–8.
3. Davis W, Porteous M. Joint replacement in the overweight patient: a logical approach or new form of rationing? Ann R Coll Surg Engl. 2007;89(3):203–6; discussion.
4. Horan F. Obesity and joint replacement. J BoneJoint Surg Br. 2006; 88(10):1269–71.
5. Santaguida PL, Hawker GA, Hudak PL, Glazier R, Mahomed NN, Kreder HJ, et al. Patient characteristics affecting the prognosis of total hip and knee joint arthroplasty: a systematic review. Can J Surg. 2008;51(6):428–36.

6. White RH, Henderson MC. Risk factors for venous thromboembolism after total hip and knee replacement surgery. Curr Opin Pulm Med. 2002;8(5):365–71.

7. Jain NB, Guller U, Pietrobon R, Bond TK, Higgins LD. Comorbidities increase complication rates in patients having arthroplasty. Clin Orthop Relat Res. 2005;435:232–8.

8. Jamsen E, Nevalainen P, Eskelinen A, Huotari K, Kalliovalkama J, Moilanen T. Obesity, diabetes, and preoperative hyperglycemia as predictors of periprosthetic joint infection: a single-center analysis of 7181 primary hip and knee replacements for osteoarthritis. J Bone Joint Surg Am. 2012;94(14):e101.

9. Miric A, Lim M, Kahn B, Rozenthal T, Bombick D, Sculco TP. Perioperative morbidity following total knee arthroplasty among obese patients. J Knee Surg. 2002;15(2):77–83.

10. Andrew JG, Palan J, Kurup HV, Gibson P, Murray DW, Beard DJ. Obesity in total hip replacement. J Bone Joint Surg Br. 2008;90(4): 424–9.

11. McCalden RW, Charron KD, Macdonald SJ, Bourne RB, Naudie DD. Does morbid obesity affect the outcome of total hip replacement?: an analysis of 3290 THRs. J Bone Joint Surg Br. 2011;93(3):321–5.

12. Jarvenpaa J, Kettunen J, Kroger H, Miettinen H. Obesity may impair the early outcome of total knee arthroplasty. Scand J Surg. 2010;99(1): 45–9.

13. Kerkhoffs GM, Servien E, Dunn W, Dahm D, Bramer JA, Haverkamp D. The influence of obesity on the complication rate and outcome of total knee arthroplasty: a meta-analysis and systematic literature review. J Bone Joint Surg Am. 2012;94(20):1839–44.

14. Hamoui N, Kantor S, Vince K, Crookes PF. Long-term outcome of total knee replacement: does obesity matter? Obes Surg. 2006;16(1): 35–8.

15. Jiganti JJ, Goldstein WM, Williams CS. A comparison of the perioperative morbidity in total joint arthroplasty in the obese and non-obese patient. Clin Orthop Relat Res. 1993;289:175–9.

16. McLaughlin JR, Lee KR. The outcome of total hip replacement in obese and non-obese patients at 10- to 18-years. J Bone Joint Surg Br. 2006;88(10):1286–92.

17. Bordini B, Stea S, Cremonini S, Viceconti M, De Palma R, Toni A. Relationship between obesity and early failure of total knee prostheses. BMC Musculoskelet Disord. 2009;10:29.

18. Amin AK, Patton JT, Cook RE, Brenkel IJ. Does obesity influence the clinical outcome at five years following total knee replacement for osteoarthritis? J Bone Joint Surg Br. 2006;88(3):335–40.

19. Chee YH, Teoh KH, Sabnis BM, Ballantyne JA, Brenkel IJ. Total hip replacement in morbidly obese patients with osteoarthritis: results of a prospectively matched study. J Bone Joint Surg Br. 2010;92(8):1066–71.

20. Bennett D, Gibson D, O'Brien S, Beverland DE. Hip arthroplasty in morbidly obese patients – intra-operative and short term outcomes. Hip Int. 2010;20(1):75–80.

21. Samson AJ, Mercer GE, Campbell DG. Total knee replacement in the morbidly obese: a literature review. ANZ J Surg. 2010;80(9):595–9.

22. Namba RS, Paxton L, Fithian DC, Stone ML. Obesity and perioperative morbidity in total hip and total knee arthroplasty patients. J Arthroplasty. 2005;20(7 Suppl 3):46–50.

23. Rajgopal V, Bourne RB, Chesworth BM, MacDonald SJ, McCalden RW, Rorabeck CH. The impact of morbid obesity on patient outcomes after total knee arthroplasty. J Arthroplasty. 2008;23(6):795–800.

24. Hamlin BR. Treatment of knee arthrosis in the morbidly obese patient. Orthop Clin North Am. 2011;42(1):107–13, vii.

25. Dewan A, Bertolusso R, Karastinos A, Conditt M, Noble PC, Parsley BS. Implant durability and knee function after total knee arthroplasty in the morbidly obese patient. J Arthroplasty. 2009;24(6 Suppl):89–94. e1–3.

26. Krushell RJ, Fingeroth RJ. Primary total knee arthroplasty in morbidly obese patients: a 5- to 14-year follow-up study. J Arthroplasty. 2007;22 (6 Suppl 2):77–80.

27. Amin AK, Clayton RA, Patton JT, Gaston M, Cook RE, Brenkel IJ. Total knee replacement in morbidly obese patients. Results of a prospective, matched study. J Bone Joint Surg Br. 2006;88(10):1321–6.

28. Winiarsky R, Barth P, Lotke P. Total knee arthroplasty in morbidly obese patients. J Bone Joint Surg Am. 1998;80(12):1770–4.

29. Pritchett JW, Bortel DT. Knee replacement in morbidly obese women. Surg Gynecol Obstet. 1991;173(2):119–22.

30. Nunez M, Lozano L, Nunez E, Sastre S, Luis Del Val J, Suso S. Good quality of life in severely obese total knee replacement patients: a case–control study. Obes Surg. 2011;21(8):1203–8.

31. Pearse EO, Caldwell BF, Lockwood RJ, Hollard J. Early mobilisation after conventional knee replacement may reduce the risk of postoperative venous thromboembolism. J Bone Joint Surg Br. 2007; 89(3):316–22. PubMed PMID: 17356141. eng.

32. Buddhdev P, Davies N, Waters TS. Obesity and the outcome of lower limb arthroplasty patients enrolled in an enhanced recovery programme: a 1000 patient study. Barcelona: World Congress on Debates and Consensus in Bone, Muscle and Joint Disease; 2012.

33. Kessler S, Kafer W. Overweight and obesity: two predictors for worse early outcome in total hip replacement? Obesity (Silver Spring). 2007;15(11):2840–5.

34. Batsis JA, Naessens JM, Keegan MT, Huddleston PM, Wagie AE, Huddleston JM. Body mass index and the impact on hospital resource use in patients undergoing total knee arthroplasty. J Arthroplasty. 2010;25(8):1250–7.e1.

35. Jenkins PJ, Clement ND, Hamilton DF, Gaston P, Patton JT, Howie CR. Predicting the cost-effectiveness of total hip and knee replacement: a health economic analysis. Bone Joint J. 2013;95-B(1):115–21.

36. Chan CL, Villar RN. Obesity and quality of life after primary hip arthroplasty. J Bone Joint Surg Br. 1996;78(1):78–81.
37. Yeung E, Jackson M, Sexton S, Walter W, Zicat B, Walter W. The effect of obesity on the outcome of hip and knee arthroplasty. Int Orthop. 2011;35(6):929–34.
38. McQueen DA, Long MJ, Algotar AM, Schurman 2nd JR, Bangalore VG. The effect of obesity on quality-of-life improvement after total knee arthroplasty. Am J Orthop (Belle Mead NJ). 2007;36(8):E117–20, E27.
39. Parvizi J, Trousdale RT, Sarr MG. Total joint arthroplasty in patients surgically treated for morbid obesity. J Arthroplasty. 2000;15(8):1003–8.
40. Sawalha S, Ravikumar R, Chowdhury EA, Massraf A. The effect of obesity on blood metal ion levels after hip resurfacing and metal-on-metal total hip replacement. Hip Int. 2012;22(1):107–12.
41. Lubbeke A, Garavaglia G, Barea C, Roussos C, Stern R, Hoffmeyer P. Influence of obesity on femoral osteolysis five and ten years following total hip arthroplasty. J Bone Joint Surg Am. 2010;92(10):1964–72.
42. Wendelboe AM, Hegmann KT, Biggs JJ, Cox CM, Portmann AJ, Gildea JH, et al. Relationships between body mass indices and surgical replacements of knee and hip joints. Am J Prev Med. 2003;25(4):290–5.
43. Kreder HJ. Review: moderate weight loss improves functional disability but does not reduce pain in obese patients with knee osteoarthritis. ACP J Club. 2007;147(2):43.
44. Christensen R, Bartels EM, Astrup A, Bliddal H. Effect of weight reduction in obese patients diagnosed with knee osteoarthritis: a systematic review and meta-analysis. Ann Rheum Dis. 2007;66(4):433–9.
45. Huang MH, Chen CH, Chen TW, Weng MC, Wang WT, Wang YL. The effects of weight reduction on the rehabilitation of patients with knee osteoarthritis and obesity. Arthritis Care Res. 2000;13(6):398–405.
46. Paans N, van den Akker-Scheek I, Dilling RG, Bos M, van der Meer K, Bulstra SK, et al. Effect of exercise and weight loss in people who have hip osteoarthritis and are overweight or obese: a prospective cohort study. Phys Ther. 2013;93(2):137–46.
47. Aderinto J, Brenkel IJ, Chan P. Weight change following total hip replacement: a comparison of obese and non-obese patients. Surgeon. 2005;3(4):305–72.
48. Lachiewicz AM, Lachiewicz PF. Weight and activity change in overweight and obese patients after primary total knee arthroplasty. J Arthroplasty. 2008;23(1):33–40.
49. Dowsey MM, Liew D, Stoney JD, Choong PF. The impact of pre-operative obesity on weight change and outcome in total knee replacement: a prospective study of 529 consecutive patients. J Bone Joint Surg Br. 2010;92(4):513–20.
50. Severson EP, Singh JA, Browne JA, Trousdale RT, Sarr MG, Lewallen DG. Total knee arthroplasty in morbidly obese patients treated with bariatric surgery: a comparative study. JArthroplasty. 2012;27(9):1696–700.

Chapter 25
Is It Time to Rename Obesity Management as Secondary Prevention?

Matthew S. Capehorn

Critics often suggest that treating obesity, in an obesogenic environment, is a waste of time, as any weight loss will return. However, obesity is a chronic relapsing condition, and whether it is due to genetics, learned behavior, society, or a mixture, it has to be accepted that some people have a predisposition to weight regain. However, morbidity and mortality are dependent on weight at any given time, and those who have undertaken weight loss programs will be at a lower weight at any given time than those who have not, even if their weight slowly creeps back on, and are therefore at lower risk of comorbidities. Obesity is associated with causing, or aggravating, over 50 common medical conditions, including important life-threatening conditions such as diabetes and cardiovascular disease, obstructive sleep apnea and other respiratory conditions, and many cancers. Rather than treat the consequences of these conditions, we should focus our attention on dealing with the cause.

M.S. Capehorn, BMedSci, MBChB
Rotherham Institute for Obesity (RIO),
Clifton Medical Centre, Doncaster Gate,
Rotherham, South Yorkshire S65 1DA, UK
e-mail: mcapehorn@yahoo.co.uk

D.W. Haslam et al. (eds.), *Controversies in Obesity*,
DOI 10.1007/978-1-4471-2834-2_25,
© Springer-Verlag London 2014

201

Prevention or Treatment

Common sense would suggest a need to focus on prevention; however, the evidence base for effective preventative measures does not exist. The discussion as to whether we need a "nanny state" or "nudge" tactics is a valid one. Many people oppose a nanny state out of principle, and a "nudge" towards healthy behavior can be very effective (e.g., an attractive staircase in your field of view may entice you away from seeking a lift or escalator). The obesogenic environment can be changed but requires the will, suitable planning, and sufficient resources.

Many different proposals have been made to help manage obesity by prevention, but will they work? A proposed 20 % fat tax will not cure the obesity problem. It makes no sense to tax fat in isolation, ignoring other food groups such as sugar. "There is no such thing as a bad food" is true in this context, as an individual can eat high-fat/high-sugar foods occasionally as part of a nutritionally balanced calorie-controlled diet. Any tax on food will therefore penalize the poor and discriminate against those of normal weight. It may not even have the desired effect of changing eating patterns (e.g., if craving a chocolate bar, a patient would pay a subsidy possibly greater than 20 % at a vending machine). Ultimately, it does not educate the patient on healthy eating or lifestyle change. Because there is no such thing as a bad food, many weight management clinics do not propose a specific "diet" that many patients find it difficult to adhere to. Instead they focus on small, achievable, and, more importantly, sustainable changes in the existing diet that have the overall effect of reducing calorie consumption and overall health improvements.

A subsidy on healthy foods, such as fruit and vegetables, may help promote "5-a-day." However, without education, this could result in additional calorie consumption. Studies, including INTERHEART [1], show that abdominal obesity is a more important modifiable risk factor for myocardial infarction that diet, and so overconsumption of even "healthy" foods, may be harmful. A meal from a "takeaway" or quick-service restaurant

(QSR) can be eaten as part of a nutritionally balanced calorie-controlled diet. The important factor is to ensure that sufficient choice is available, to allow the consumer a "healthy" alternative, and to not, for example, place a row of QSRs outside a school. A sensible proposal would be to restrict portion sizes served by QSRs, as recently proposed by Mayor Bloomberg in New York, and to further encourage calorie information on menus, which is being made standard by the National Restaurant Association, in conjunction with the limitation of unnecessary, inappropriate advertising targeting children.

Other preventative measures may be worth implementing, based upon "sensible assumptions" rather than a body of evidence to support them. For example, the school curriculum should include health and well-being, including specific education on obesity, its importance, effects on the body and consequences, social impact, etc., as well as teaching of correct portion sizes, knowledge about calories, cooking, benefits of physical activity, knowledge of local services available, etc. Furthermore, as Jamie Oliver demonstrated in Rotherham, in his "Ministry of Food" television program, there are many people that do not have basic cooking skills, such as being able to boil an egg. It is futile for weight management service providers to educate on the benefits of cooking from raw ingredients if patients then go home without the skills. All weight management services should work in partnership with teams that can deliver cooking skills.

The Health-Economic Argument

At present, considerably more money is invested in the prevention of obesity than its management [2]. Some estimate that £5bn has been invested in prevention and yet only £30m on treatment [3, 4]. Health-economic data suggest that focusing all resources on prevention may not be the most cost-effective strategy [2]. Foresight proposed that a preventative intervention may be as costly as doing nothing. However, there is evidence that treatment interventions work, conveying significant health-economic benefits. Furthermore, obesity management should be considered as *secondary prevention*, as we do with cardiovascular disease. In this sense, the management of the obese prevents further obesity, morbid obesity, the super-obese, and so on. This management should take place in the primary care setting.

Barriers to Effective Obesity Management

Barriers to weight management services may be found within the health care profession, with patients and their relationship with the professional, or be organizational – lack of sufficiently resourced and funded services.

In the UK, incentivizing GPs to focus attention on obesity is achievable through the existing Quality and Outcomes Framework (QOF), which represents the performance-related pay element to a GP's income. At present, the only QOF indicator that directly targets obesity rewards GPs for registering the number of obese people that they see. Merely drawing a register will not prevent a single overweight person from developing type 2 diabetes or a single obese person from having a heart attack.

Recent debate has surrounded use of the word "obesity." It is true that in certain circumstances, referring to a patient "not being at a healthy weight" may be preferable, but it must not be ignored that the word "obesity" carries important beneficial connotations (e.g., a parent of an obese child may insist they did not have to worry about their child's weight because their school letter said they were only "very overweight" or "not at a healthy weight" instead of referring to him/her as "obese"). The parent may understand the importance of obesity and would ask for help if their child was obese but not be concerned without the use of that term.

Further recent debate has surrounded whether overweight doctors, or other health care professionals, are less likely to give diet and lifestyle advice to their patients or be as effective in delivering this information [5]. Health care professionals are only human and can lead unhealthy lifestyles as well as their patients, but does it make them less successful at delivering healthy lifestyle messages? If a doctor smokes, does it affect their ability to give effective smoking cessation advice? If a doctor drinks over the recommended amount of alcohol each week, does it affect their ability to give effective alcohol consumption advice? However, one problem may be that if a doctor smokes or drinks too much, this may not be evident to the patient. If a doctor is overweight/obese, this will be noticed, and although they may be able to give good advice to the patient, how will it be received?

Some health care professionals lack the skills to raise the issue of weight with appropriate subtle brief interventions and motivational interviewing techniques, or it may be that the patient (or the parent, in the case of an overweight child) does not have the desire to raise the issue or the motivation to do anything about their weight even if there is acceptance of it. Thus, *motivation* may be a key barrier to engagement with services. Patients sent to a weight management clinic, directly from a chronic disease clinic assessment purely because of their weight, may not be as successful as those patients who present raising the issue of their own weight and expressing a desire to tackle it. This may in part explain why there is a different response of patients enrolled in clinical weight loss trials to those in real-life practice. It is vital that in the situation in which an individual expresses motivation to reach a more healthy weight that suitable weight management services are available locally.

There should be investment in structured frameworks, to help provide local areas with integrated interventions at all levels, such as the award-winning NHS Rotherham Healthy Weights Framework (Fig. 25.1) in Yorkshire, England. Investment should be long-term (10 years+) rather than as short-term commissions to providers, which currently inhibits service development. Albeit based on crude extrapolation of costs for the NHS Rotherham Framework, similar services could be developed to cover the UK for an estimated £240m per year [6] (considerably less than the government's anticipated direct and indirect costs of obesity).

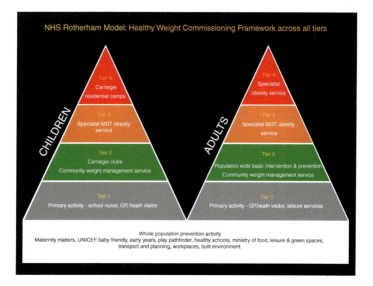

FIGURE 25.1   The NHS Rotherham Obesity Healthy Weight Framework for the management of healthy weight in adults and children

This structured framework approach to weight management, including a comprehensive multidisciplinary team, as well as community weight management programs, needs to be encouraged and developed. Tier 4 interventions such as bariatric surgery in adults are cost-effective [7] but only in appropriate patients. Weight loss surgery does not "make" someone thin, as the media portray, but may allow someone to feel satiated on an eggcup full of food. Unfortunately, surgery itself does not control what *type of food* is consumed (including calories from liquids or foods digested within 20 min rendering surgery less effective), or provide the *willpower* to avoid over-frequent "eggcups" full of food, or address any underlying *emotional eating* issues that result in comfort eating or habit eating and that will persist after surgery unless sufficient talking therapies have been delivered, before and after surgery. This psychological support is highlighted as being as important as the surgery itself [8]. More expensive interventions will only be effective as part of a framework of interventions that allows for the proper assessment and triage of appropriate patients for the most appropriate treatment, which is best done in a primary care setting. The surgical operation is a brief technological interlude in a program that starts the moment a patient is identified and engaged and ends on the death of the individual, hopefully at age 93 in a snowboarding accident. This program is almost entirely undertaken within the realm of primary care.

The NHS Rotherham Obesity Strategy

The NHS Rotherham Healthy Weight Framework won the 2009 NHS Health and Social Care Award for excellence in commissioning. Funding has been made available to continue the services, based on proven success and health-economic arguments. Total cost for all interventions is currently approximately £1m per year for the population of Rotherham, which is just in excess of 250,000.

The framework involves four levels of intervention:

The initial level of intervention is the activity most often done in the primary care setting, which involves identifying those patients that have weight problems and who are *motivated to change*, especially those with medical conditions that are likely to worsen with increasing weight. It is important to clarify that this primary activity, and any associated health promotion advice, can be delivered by any health care professional from primary or secondary care or in the pharmacy, council, leisure services, or private sector.

The second tier of intervention is a community-based, time-limited, weight management program of diet, nutrition, lifestyle, and exercise advice delivered by trained staff. For adults, this is the Reshape Rotherham program delivered by the Rotherham dietetics department, and for children, this is the *More Life* (formerly Carnegie) *Clubs* program. Patients can be referred, or self-refer, to these services.

Patients who do not meet their healthy weight targets in this level of intervention, or those who are considered to be more at risk of comorbidities and/or require more specialist intervention, are referred into the third tier, which is the specialist service delivered by the Rotherham Institute for Obesity (RIO), which has a *multidisciplinary team approach* to managing weight problems by providing specialists that can provide different approaches (Table 25.1). Patients are

TABLE 25.1 Summary of facilities offered at RIO

Job description	Role
Health trainers	Brief interventions and motivational interviewing
	Goal setting and life-coaching
Health care assistant	Weighing and measuring
	Follow-up care
	VLCD monitoring
	OSA screening
Obesity specialist nurse	Initial triage
	Basic nutrition and advice
	VLCD initiation
	OSA screening
Dietitian	Complex dietary needs including VLCD support
	Pre-/post-op bariatric surgery
"Cook and eat"	Basic nutrition and advice
	Cooking skills (on-site kitchen facilities)
Exercise therapists	Personal exercise program (on-site gym)
	Education and motivation
	Liaison with other local physical activity events/sites
Talking therapists	Life-coaching
	Cognitive behavioral therapy (CBT)
	Neurolinguistic programming (NLP)
	Emotional freedom techniques (EFT)
GPWSI	Pharmacotherapy
	Pre-bariatric surgery and pre-residential camp assessments
	OSA referrals

TABLE 25.1 (continued)

Job description	Role
Admin. supervisor	Liaison with patients, referrers, and other service providers
	Allocation of appointments
Clinical manager	Managing service and clinical governance
Education room/ library	Resource room; group work
Bariatric surgery center	Potential for bariatric intragastric balloons (BIB) and endobarriers
	Potential for overnight sleep studies
Other specialists	Obstetric preconception care, e.g.
RIO market stall	Advice at the point of sale of fruit and vegetables
	Promotion of healthy weight framework services

required to be assessed by RIO before they can access any tier 4 services, such as bariatric surgery in the case of adults or residential weight management camps (delivered by More Life, formerly Carnegie) in the case of children.

References

1. Yusuf S, Hawken S, Ounpuu S, Dans T, Avezum A, Lanas F, et al. Effect of potentially modifiable risk factors associated with myocardial infarction in 52 countries (the INTERHEART study). Lancet. 2004;364:9437.
2. HM treasury public spending review 2010. Cm7492. London: Stationery Office, 6. 2010.
3. Gately P. Childhood obesity. Oral presentation. ASO Conference: lightening the load in primary care. University College, London. 2012.
4. Sacher P. Child obesity: problems and solutions. Oral presentation. Obesity 2012 Conference: the management of obesity and its complications. Hallam Conference Centre, London. 2012.
5. Bleich SN, Bennett WL, Gudzune KA, Cooper LA, et al. Impact of physician BMI on obesity care and beliefs. Obesity (Silver Spring). 2012;20(5):999–1005.

6. Capehorn M. RIO: the MDT approach to tackling obesity. Oral presentation. National obesity forum Conference. Royal College of Physicians, London. 2012.
7. Shedding the pounds: obesity management, NICE guidance and bariatric surgery in England. London: Office of Health Economics. 2010. Available from: http://www.rcseng.ac.uk/news/docs/BariatricReport.pdf.
8. Too lean a service: a review of the care of patients that underwent bariatric surgery. National confidential enquiry into patient outcome and death. 2012. Available from: http://www.ncepod.org.uk/2012report2/downloads/BS_fullreport.pdf.

Part V
Childhood

Chapter 26
Childhood Obesity: What Harm, Any Solutions?

Julian Paul Hamilton-Shield

The latest and most reliable figures for childhood obesity in England come from the National Child Measurement Programme (NCMP), which has a coverage of approximately 93 % of reception (aged 5 years) and year-6 (aged 11 years) children [1]. By the time children leave primary school, 19 % are obese and 14 % overweight. With over a third of children overweight or obese at 11 years, it is more than worrying that both adiposity and cardiovascular risk demonstrate at least moderate tracking into adult life [2, 3]. Encouragingly, on a population basis there is evidence that positively changing weight status from around primary school-leaving age through late adolescence has a beneficial effect on later cardiovascular risk [4] and thus interventions aimed at improving weight status in childhood seem an entirely appropriate public health goal. However, broad-scale, population-based interventions are hampered by an inability of both health professionals [5] and families [6, 7] to recognize obesity in those they meet or care for, probably due to the general upward trend in adiposity witnessed over the last 20 years.

J.P. Hamilton-Shield, MBChB, MD
NIHR Biomedical Research Unit in Nutrition and Bristol,
Royal Hospital for Children, University of Bristol,
Upper Maudlin Street, Bristol, BS28AE, UK
e-mail: j.p.h.shield@bristol.ac.uk

D.W. Haslam et al. (eds.), *Controversies in Obesity*,
DOI 10.1007/978-1-4471-2834-2_26,
© Springer-Verlag London 2014

213

Furthermore, despite numerous media headlines and governmental initiatives, there is still a significant section of society that seems inured and unwilling to accept the basic health message that obesity, including that in childhood, is bad for health [8, 9]. In financial terms, it is currently difficult to estimate the direct economic burden of childhood obesity [10], but the Foresight report on the projected NHS costs of overweight and obesity in general makes for sobering reading (£9.7 billion by 2050) [11].

For the clinician, it is probably more pertinent for patient and family engagement in addressing clinical obesity to consider the effects of obesity on an individual basis. While it is undoubtedly the case that childhood obesity is most likely to have overt health repercussions in adult life, which makes therapy in childhood a hard sell to many families, there is evidence of significant harm in numerous individuals presenting to childhood obesity clinics. Idiopathic intracranial hypertension [12], nonalcoholic steatohepatitis [13], orthopedic problems [14], sleep-disordered breathing [15], and type 2 diabetes [16] have all been documented in association with childhood/adolescent obesity. Type 2 diabetes is a good example of the potential impact of childhood obesity on long-term health. While in the UK it is still far less common than type 1 diabetes in childhood [17], such a diagnosis in adolescence will likely have profound implications for longevity and health [18]. There is evidence that such complications as diabetic nephropathy are more prevalent in type 2 diabetes developing in young people than the traditional childhood illness of type 1 diabetes [19, 20]. In addition, self-esteem in the young with weight problems is low [21, 22] and likely lower if complicated by diabetes. This probably accounts for the notoriously poor compliance [23] and high dropout levels from clinics [24] that make effective therapy very difficult to deliver. In addition, it is worth considering the considerable impact of obesity and type 2 diabetes in early adult life. The rising prevalence of pregnancy-associated obesity in young adult women and the closely associated companion, poorly controlled type 2 diabetes is undoubtedly placing additional burden on the individual mothers but also on their offspring in terms of infant mortality and morbidity and later childhood metabolic health [25]. The surest method to stem the rise of perinatal, obesity-related disease is to address obesity in childhood and not wait for interventions from the antenatal booking clinic onward.

Thus, if there is a legitimate case to consider childhood obesity a public and individual threat to future health, what interventions should be considered? In the community setting, while the National Child Measurement Programme data are not routinely fed back to primary care physicians, there is an argument for fiscal remuneration to general practice for collecting and acting upon simple measures of adiposity for children and adolescents. Currently, there is a degree of ambivalence towards primary care management of childhood obesity [26], and data collection on most children does not extend to a measurement of weight or body mass index [27]. Encouraging an emphasis on healthy weight in primary care for all children would be a step forward. Social policies to encourage healthier eating should also be adopted. While healthy eating is not necessarily economically prohibitive for the majority of families [28], it could and has been argued that taxing energy-dense food and drink, such as recently happened in Denmark [29], would be progressive as opposed to regressive tax liable to improve the long-term health of the economically disadvantaged [30].

For the individual obese child, two aspects need consideration: the extent of overweight or obesity and evidence of secondary comorbidities. There is currently a dearth of evidence demonstrating that simple behavior interventions aimed at increasing physical activity and improving healthy eating have a significant clinical impact on levels of adiposity [31]. It is pertinent to point out that the lack of evidence does not reflect the myriad of interventions trialled. Consequently, there is a need to explore alternative avenues for intervention. Areas that probably may prove beneficial as adjuncts to simple physical activity and nutrition change interventions include addressing eating behaviors and taste preferences. We recently published data suggesting that training obese children to eat more slowly improved their ability to recognize satiety and, thus, portion size decreased, as did BMI SDS scores. Furthermore, weight improvement was sustained post-intervention, suggesting a level of behavioral imprinting [32].

For those individual children with very significant obesity simply categorized as a BMI >40 kg/m^2 or those with comorbidities and BMI >35, interventions should be tailored to address the seriousness of the condition. In general, pharmacological resources for the treatment of childhood obesity are few and usually of limited value [33]. A randomized trial of bariatric surgery (laparoscopic gastric banding) versus standard medical management of severe adolescent obesity documented far greater weight loss and greatly improved remission from metabolic syndrome in those having surgery [34]. Furthermore, cases for surgery can be made on an individual basis in those with significant health consequences attendant or worsened by their adiposity [35, 36] Recently, publications from both the USA and the UK have drawn attention to the possible need to consider state intervention in the form of child safeguarding and foster placement for some children in whom all efforts to address obesity in the home setting have failed, with significant increasing of weight in the face of intensive lifestyle interventions together with apparent failure of parental engagement [37, 38].

Conclusion

The UK and most other developed and developing countries in the world are facing unprecedented levels of childhood obesity. Strategies to encourage improved societal awareness of the consequences require urgent development to reduce overall prevalence. On an individual basis, interventions need tailoring to the levels of obesity and associated comorbidities. While the majority of children should respond to simple lifestyle interventions that may need a broader focus than physical activity and healthy diet alone, obesity in more severe cases does require far greater resources medically, socially, and politically.

Acknowledgement   JPHS is supported by an NIHR Biomedical Research Unit in Nutrition award to University Hospitals Bristol NHS Foundation Trust. The views expressed in this publication are those of the author and not necessarily those of the NHS, the National Institute for Health Research or the Department of Health.

References

1. The NHS Information Centre LS. National child measurement programme. London: The NHS Information Centre LS; 2011.
2. Herman KM, Craig CL, Gauvin L, Katzmarzyk PT. Tracking of obesity and physical activity from childhood to adulthood: the Physical Activity Longitudinal Study. Int J Pediatr Obes. 2009;4(4):281–8.
3. Singh AS, Mulder C, Twisk JW, van Mechelen W, Chinapaw MJ. Tracking of childhood overweight into adulthood: a systematic review of the literature. Obes Rev. 2008;9(5):474–88.
4. Lawlor DA, Benfield L, Logue J, Tilling K, Howe LD, Fraser A, et al. Association between general and central adiposity in childhood, and change in these, with cardiovascular risk factors in adolescence: prospective cohort study. BMJ. 2010;341:c6224.
5. Smith SM, Gately P, Rudolf M. Can we recognise obesity clinically? Arch Dis Child. 2008;93(12):1065–6.
6. Carnell S, Edwards C, Croker H, Boniface D, Wardle J. Parental perceptions of overweight in 3–5 y olds. Int J Obes (Lond). 2005;29(4):353–5.
7. Parry LL, Netuveli G, Parry J, Saxena S. A systematic review of parental perception of overweight status in children. J Ambul Care Manage. 2008;31(3):253–68.
8. Eckstein KC, Mikhail LM, Ariza AJ, Thomson JS, Millard SC, Binns HJ. Parents' perceptions of their child's weight and health. Pediatrics. 2006;117(3):681–90.
9. Lampard AM, Byrne SM, Zubrick SR, Davis EA. Parents' concern about their children's weight. Int J Pediatr Obes. 2008;3(2):84–92.
10. John J, Wolfenstetter SB, Wenig CM. An economic perspective on childhood obesity: recent findings on cost of illness and cost effectiveness of interventions. Nutrition. 2012;28(9):829–39.
11. Kopelman P, Jebb SA, Butland B. Executive summary: foresight 'tackling obesities: future choices' project. Obes Rev. 2007;8 Suppl 1:vi–ix.
12. Brara SM, Koebnick C, Porter AH, Langer-Gould A. Pediatric idiopathic intracranial hypertension and extreme childhood obesity. J Pediatr. 2012;161(4):602–7.
13. Wei C, Ford A, Hunt L, Crowne EC, Shield JP. Abnormal liver function in children with metabolic syndrome from a UK-based obesity clinic. Arch Dis Child. 2011;96(11):1003–7.

14. Lifshitz F. Obesity in children. J Clin Res Pediatr Endocrinol. 2008;1(2):53–60.
15. Wing YK, Hui SH, Pak WM, Ho CK, Cheung A, Li AM, et al. A controlled study of sleep related disordered breathing in obese children. Arch Dis Child. 2003;88(12):1043–7.
16. Haines L, Wan KC, Lynn R, Barrett TG, Shield JP. Rising incidence of type 2 diabetes in children in the U.K. Diabetes Care. 2007;30(5): 1097–101.
17. National Paediatric Diabetes Audit Project Board, Royal College of Paediatrics and Child Health. National Paediatric Diabetes Audit Report 2009/10. http://www.hqip.org.uk/assets/NCAPOP-Library/NHSIC-National-Diabetes-Paediatric-Audit-Report-2009-2010.pdf.
18. Kavey RE, Allada V, Daniels SR, Hayman LL, McCrindle BW, Newburger JW, et al. Cardiovascular risk reduction in high-risk pediatric patients: a scientific statement from the American Heart Association Expert Panel on Population and Prevention Science; the Councils on Cardiovascular Disease in the Young, Epidemiology and Prevention, Nutrition, Physical Activity and Metabolism, High Blood Pressure Research, Cardiovascular Nursing, and the Kidney in Heart Disease; and the Interdisciplinary Working Group on Quality of Care and Outcomes Research: endorsed by the American Academy of Pediatrics. Circulation. 2006;114(24):2710–38.
19. Maahs DM, Snively BM, Bell RA, Dolan L, Hirsch I, Imperatore G, et al. Higher prevalence of elevated albumin excretion in youth with type 2 than type 1 diabetes: the SEARCH for Diabetes in Youth study. Diabetes Care. 2007;30(10):2593–8.
20. Svensson M, Sundkvist G, Arnqvist HJ, Bjork E, Blohme G, Bolinder J, et al. Signs of nephropathy may occur early in young adults with diabetes despite modern diabetes management: results from the nationwide population-based Diabetes Incidence Study in Sweden (DISS). Diabetes Care. 2003;26(10):2903–9.
21. Wang F, Veugelers PJ. Self-esteem and cognitive development in the era of the childhood obesity epidemic. Obes Rev. 2008;9(6):615–23.
22. Wang F, Wild TC, Kipp W, Kuhle S, Veugelers PJ. The influence of childhood obesity on the development of self-esteem. Health Rep. 2009;20(2):21–7.
23. Shield JP, Lynn R, Wan KC, Haines L, Barrett TG. Management and 1 year outcome for UK children with type 2 diabetes. Arch Dis Child. 2009;94(3):206–9.
24. Reinehr T, Schober E, Roth CL, Wiegand S, Holl R. Type 2 diabetes in children and adolescents in a 2-year follow-up: insufficient adherence to diabetes centers. Horm Res. 2008;69(2):107–13.
25. Temple R, Murphy H. Type 2 diabetes in pregnancy – an increasing problem. Best Pract Res Clin Endocrinol Metab. 2010;24(4):591–603.
26. Turner KM, Shield JP, Salisbury C. Practitioners' views on managing childhood obesity in primary care: a qualitative study. Br J Gen Pract. 2009;59(568):856–62.

27. Banks J, Shield JP, Sharp D. Barriers engaging families and GPs in childhood weight management strategies. Br J Gen Pract. 2011;61(589):e492–7.
28. Banks J, Williams J, Cumberlidge T, Cimonetti T, Sharp DJ, Shield JP. Is healthy eating for obese children necessarily more costly for families? Br J Gen Pract. 2012;62(594):e1–5.
29. Wilkins R. Danes impose 25% tax increases on ice cream, chocolate, and sweets to curb disease. BMJ. 2010;341:c3592.
30. Mytton OT, Clarke D, Rayner M. Taxing unhealthy food and drinks to improve health. BMJ. 2012;344:e2931.
31. Oude Luttikhuis H, Baur L, Jansen H, Shrewsbury VA, O'Malley C, Stolk RP, et al. Interventions for treating obesity in children. Cochrane Database Syst Rev. 2009;(1):CD001872.
32. Ford AL, Bergh C, Sodersten P, Sabin MA, Hollinghurst S, Hunt LP, et al. Treatment of childhood obesity by retraining eating behaviour: randomised controlled trial. BMJ. 2010;340:b5388.
33. Sabin MA, Magnussen CG, Juonala M, Cowley MA, Shield JP. The role of pharmacotherapy in the prevention and treatment of paediatric metabolic syndrome–implications for long-term health: part of a series on Pediatric Pharmacology, guest edited by Gianvincenzo Zuccotti, Emilio Clementi, and Massimo Molteni. Pharmacol Res. 2012;65(4):397–401.
34. O'Brien PE, Sawyer SM, Laurie C, Brown WA, Skinner S, Veit F, et al. Laparoscopic adjustable gastric banding in severely obese adolescents: a randomized trial. JAMA. 2010;303(6):519–26.
35. Shield JP, Crowne E, Morgan J. Is there a place for bariatric surgery in treating childhood obesity? Arch Dis Child. 2008;93(5):369–72.
36. Daskalakis M, Till H, Kiess W, Weiner RA. Roux-en-Y gastric bypass in an adolescent patient with Bardet-Biedl syndrome, a monogenic obesity disorder. Obes Surg. 2010;20(1):121–5.
37. Viner RM, Roche E, Maguire SA, Nicholls DE. Childhood protection and obesity: framework for practice. BMJ. 2010;341:c3074.
38. Murtagh L, Ludwig DS. State intervention in life-threatening childhood obesity. JAMA. 2011;306(2):206–7.

Chapter 27
Residential Weight Loss Camps for Children and Young People

Paul J. Gately

Background

Childhood obesity has been described as the modern-day plague given the scale and its negative health consequences, prompting widespread calls for action by international [1, 2] and national [3–5] organizations.

Childhood obesity levels have increased over the last 30 years, with the most significant growth in the severe obesity range [6]. For example, Skelton et al. [7] reported a 300 % increase in severe obesity of US children from 1976 to 2004. Furthermore, UK reports outlined the greatest increase in BMI was found in children who were already overweight or obese [8].

The deleterious consequences of childhood obesity have been well documented. There is evidence that CVD risk factors in children increase exponentially with increasing BMI [9] and that the duration of obesity is a key risk factor for life expectancy [10] . In addition to these negative associations with physical health [11], childhood obesity has been linked

P.J. Gately, BA (Hons), MMedSci, PhD
Carnegie Faculty of Sport and Education,
Leeds Metropolitan University, Churchwood Hall,
Headingley Campus, Leeds, West Yorkshire LS6 3QS, UK
e-mail: p.gately@leedsmet.ac.uk

D.W. Haslam et al. (eds.), *Controversies in Obesity*,
DOI 10.1007/978-1-4471-2834-2_27,
© Springer-Verlag London 2014

221

to poorer psychological [12, 13] and social health [14] and economic well-being [15].

Childhood Obesity Treatment Options

There are a range of treatment options available for individual families and health purchasers. The most common being community programs that offer diet, physical activity, and lifestyle change. The Cochrane Review [16] reported that the degree of weight loss that can be achieved using these approaches is relatively small and, as a result, likely to be limited in reducing long-term health risks in the severely obese.

An alternative to community-based weight loss programs are intensive RWLC. Like other treatment approaches, information on diet and physical activity and behavior change are major features of these programs. The additional advantage of this approach is that they have the potential to be more holistic and spend a greater amount of time addressing broader (and probably more important) social, psychological, and emotional issues related to their obesity.

Evidence-Based Outcomes

RWLC have been delivered and evaluated in both the USA [17–20] and Europe [21–23]. These programs are typically run during the summer vacation period and last between 6 and 8 weeks. Although there is limited evidence of the effectiveness of RWLC, emerging research indicates their benefits in addressing multiple issues and superior attrition rates (6.8 % vs. 19.7 %) when compared to outpatient treatment programs [24, 25].

Weight Loss

Given that RWLC can create a highly controlled environment, significant weight loss is reported, although there is variation in the weight loss outcomes between programs. For example, Rohrbacher [18] reported losses of 13.7 kg, while Gately et al. [22]

more recently reported lower weight losses of 6 kg and 2.4 BMI units. Despite such variations, these results are much greater than those reported in community programs.

Physical Health Benefits

RWLC have been shown to induce improvements in several indices of physical health. Hobkirk et al. [26] reported significant improvements in several cardiometabolic variables, while Gately et al. [22] reported significant improvements in systolic and diastolic blood pressure and aerobic fitness. King et al. [27] showed significant reductions in improvements in LDL cholesterol with the degree of LDL peak particle size significantly increased. All demonstrated major physical health benefits.

Psychosocial Benefits

The holistic nature of RWLC has also been shown to positively influence a range of psychosocial variables. Several researchers have reported significant improvements in a range of psychological and well-being variables [18, 22, 28–30]. Several studies have reported significant improvements in global self-worth, athletic competence, and physical appearance. Barton [29] reported significant improvements in cognitive changes in diet and physical activity behaviors during a 6-week RWLC.

Holt et al. [31] reported positive experiences in the form of enjoyment, peer support, as well as staff support and a choice of activities. Holt found that slightly under half of the participants in the study reported bullying concerns prior to the program, but that they did not experience any bullying.

Follow-Up

The long-term outcomes of RWLC are an important question. Gately et al. [32] reported that 89 % of participants had maintained their weight or lost more at 1-year follow-up. Hester et al. [33], using a qualitative methodology, reported positive long-term outcomes at 6 and 12 months, with further weight loss or weight loss maintenance, and the enjoyment of diet and physical activity behaviors. Beyond weight loss and the adoption of new lifestyle behaviors, other important and relevant long-term impacts to the children's lives included the wearing of new styles of clothes, improvements in school engagement, and making new friends. Hester also reported a series of challenges that warrant further research. These include conflicting messages from family, friends, and medical practitioners.

Quality Care

As with all health interventions, quality care and clinical governance are critical to ensure effective outcomes. Unfortunately, many RWLC do not fit within any health-care monitoring framework, and practices vary widely. Many of the non-expert-led programs have a "boot camp" approach, which is not in line with a positive motivational climate that is necessary to engage young people in long-term behavior change [34]. There is clearly a need for expert-led and evidence-based approaches to ensure safe and effective practice.

Conclusion

With a high and growing prevalence of severe obesity and a broad range of negative consequences this brings, RLWC offer a valuable holistic approach to weight loss and weight loss maintenance. The short- and long-term weight loss outcomes of RWLC and their associated physical, psychological, and social benefits demonstrate their effectiveness as a treatment modality. Despite the evidence of impact and need, these interventions do not figure in national guidance on tackling obesity, which tends to be dominated by primary preventative action. In the UK, for example, it is estimated that there are 140,000 children that are three standard deviations above the norm for their weight, and yet there are only two RWLCs available, with minimal public funding. In the absence of these interventions, the likely future for severely obese children is that they will become an increasing burden on health and social care systems, and/or they will become patients of bariatric surgery at some point in adolescence or early adulthood.

References

1. WHO. Preventing and managing the global epidemic of obesity. Report of the World Health Organization. Consultation of obesity. Geneva: WHO; 1997.
2. WHO. Global strategy on diet, physical activity and health. Geneva: World Health Organisation; 2004.
3. Department of Health. Healthy weight healthy lives. London: HMSO; 2008.
4. Department of Health. Call to action: obesity strategy. London: HMSO; 2011.
5. Koplan JP, Liverman CT, Kraak VA, Committee on Prevention of Obesity in Children and Youth, Institute of Medicine, editors. Preventing childhood obesity: health in the balance. Washington, DC: The National Academies; 2004.
6. Hedley AA, Ogden CL, Johnson CL, Carroll MD, Curtin LR, Flegal KM. Prevalence of overweight and obesity among US children, adolescents, and adults, 1999–2002. JAMA. 2004;291(23):2847–50.
7. Skelton JA, Cook SR, Auinger P, Klein JD, Barlow SE. Prevalence and trends of severe obesity among US children and adolescents. Acad Pediatr. 2009;9(5):322–9. doi:10.1016/j.acap.2009.04.005#_blank.
8. National Obesity Observatory. National child measurement program: detailed analysis of the 2007/08. National Dataset, London, HM Government. Apr 2009.
9. Freedman DS, Katzmarzyk PT, Dietz WH, Srinivasan SR, Berenson GS. Relation of body mass index and skinfold thicknesses to cardiovascular disease risk factors in children: the Bogalusa Heart Study. Am J Clin Nutr. 2009;90:210–6.
10. Abdullah A, Wolfe R, Stoelwinder JU, De Courten M, Stevenson C, Walls HL, et al. The number of years lived with obesity and the risk of all-cause and cause-specific mortality. Int J Epidemiol. 2011;40:985–96.
11. Reilly JJ, Methven E, McDowell ZC, Hacking B, Alexander D, Stewart L, et al. Health consequences of obesity. Arch Dis Child. 2003;88:748–52.

12. Schwimmer JB, Burwinkle TM, Varni JW. Health related quality of life of severely obese children and adolescents. JAMA. 2003;289:1813–9.

13. Luppino FS, de Wit LM, Bouvy PF, Stijnen T, Cuijpers P, Penninx BW, et al. Overweight, obesity, and depression: a systematic review and meta-analysis of longitudinal studies. Arch Gen Psychiatry. 2010;67(3):220–9.

14. Hill AJ. Chapter 14. Social and psychological factors in obesity. In: Williams G, Frühbeck G, editors. Obesity science to practice. Chichester: Wiley; 2009. p. 347–63.

15. Glass CM, Haas SA, Reither EN. The skinny on success: body mass, gender and occupational standing across the life course. Soc Forces. 2010;88(4):1777–806.

16. Oude LH, Baur L, Jansen H, Shrewsbury VA, O'Malley C, Stolk RP, et al. Interventions for treating obesity in children (Review). Cochrane Database Syst Rev. 2009;(1):CD001872.

17. Cooper C, Sarvey S, Collier D, Willson C, Green I, Pories ML, et al. For comparison: experience with a children's obesity camp. Surg Obes Relat Dis. 2006;2:622–6.

18. Rohrbacher R. Influence of a special camp program for obese boys on weight loss, self-concept and body image. Res Q. 1973;44:150–7.

19. Gately PJ, Cooke CB, Knight C, Carroll S. The acute effects of an 8-week diet, exercise, and educational camp program on obese children. Pediatr Exerc Sci. 2000;12:413–23.

20. Huelsing J, Kanafani N, Mao J, White NH. Camp jump start: effects of a residential summer weight-loss camp for older children and adolescents. Pediatrics. 2010;125(4):e884–90.

21. Braet C, Tanghe A, Decaluwé V, Moens E, Rosseel Y. Inpatient treatment for children with obesity: weight loss, psychological well-being, and eating behavior. J Pediatr Psychol. 2004;29(7):519–29.

22. Gately PJ, Cooke CB, Barth JH, Bewick BM, Radley D, Hill AJ. Residential weight loss programs can work: a prospective cohort study of acute outcomes for overweight and obese children. Pediatrics. 2005;116:73–7.

23. Nowicka P, Lanke J, Pietrobelli A, Apitzsch E, Flodmark CE. Sports camp with six months of support from a local sports club as a treatment for childhood obesity. Scand J Public Health. 2009;37(8):793–800.

24. Kelly KP, Kirschenbaum DS. Immersion treatment of childhood and adolescent obesity: the first review of a promising intervention. Obes Rev. 2011;12(1):37–49.

25. Wilfley DE, Tibbs TL, Van Buren DJ, Reach KP, Walker MS, Epstein LH. Lifestyle interventions in the treatment of childhood overweight: a meta-analytic review of randomized controlled trials. Health Psychol. 2007;26:521–32.

26. Hobkirk JP, King RF, Gately P, Pemberton P, Smith A, Barth JH, et al. Longitudinal factor analysis reveals a distinct clustering of cardiometabolic improvements during intensive, short-term dietary

and exercise intervention in obese children and adolescents. Metab Syndr Relat Disord. 2012;10:20–5.

27. King RF, Hobkirk JP, Cooke CB, Radley D, Gately PJ. Low-density lipoprotein sub-fraction profiles in obese children before and after attending a residential weight loss intervention. J Atheroscler Thromb. 2008;15(2):100–7.

28. Braet C, VanWinckel M. Long-term follow-up of a cognitive behavioral treatment program for obese children. Behav Ther. 2000;31:55–74.

29. Barton SB, Walker LLM, Lambert G, Gately PJ, Hill AJ. Cognitive change in obese adolescents losing weight. Obes Res. 2000;12:313–9.

30. Walker LM, Gately PJ, Bewick BM, Hill AJ. Children's weight loss camps: psychological benefit or jeopardy? Int J Obes. 2003;27:748–54.

31. Holt NL, Bewick BM, Gately PJ. Children's perceptions of attending a residential weight-loss camp in the UK. Child Care Health Dev. 2005;31:223–31.

32. Gately PJ, Cooke CB, Mackreth P, Carroll S. The effects of a children's summer camp program on weight loss, with a 10-month follow-up. Int J Obes. 2000;11:1445–52.

33. Hester JR, McKenna J, Gately PJ. Obese young people's accounts of intervention impact. Patient Educ Couns. 2010;79(3):306–14.

34. Ames C. Achievement goals, motivational climate, and motivational processes. In: Roberts GC, editor. Motivation in sport and exercise. Champaign: Human Kinetics; 1992. p. 161–76.

Part VI
Treatment

Chapter 28
Sibutramine and Rimonabant: A Postmortem Forensic Examination

Gary Wittert

Sibutramine increases satiety by inhibiting the reuptake of serotonin and noradrenaline (norepinephrine), with a secondary effect on energy metabolism whereby it attenuates some of the fall in metabolic rate that follows weight loss.

The production of endocannabinoids in tissues and the levels in the circulation are increased in obesity, particularly when predominantly visceral. Rimonabant, a cannabinoid type 1 receptor antagonist, reduces weight by both central and peripheral mechanisms of action.

Both sibutramine and rimonabant produce weight loss of, on average, about 5 kg at 12 months, which is maintained at 2 years with ongoing drug use. But beyond any weight-dependent benefits, they differ in their effects, either beneficial or otherwise, for cardiovascular risk.

Both sibutramine and rimonabant have, however, now been withdrawn, and all companies have discontinued the development of drugs targeting the CB1 receptor centrally.

G. Wittert, MB Bch, MD, FRACP, FRCP
Discipline of Medicine, University of Adelaide,
L6, Eleanor Harrald Building, RAH Frome Street,
Adelaide, SA 5000, Australia
e-mail: gary.wittert@adelaide.edu.au

D.W. Haslam et al. (eds.), *Controversies in Obesity*,
DOI 10.1007/978-1-4471-2834-2_28,
© Springer-Verlag London 2014

Effects on the Cardio-metabolic Risk and Reason for Withdrawal

Sibutramine

Data from the clinical development program show that sibutramine lowers triglyceride levels, normalizes HDL, and induces variable increases in, or at least attenuates, the expected weight-loss-associated fall in diastolic blood pressure and consistently increases heart rate [1, 2].

Resting heart rate has been shown to be positively associated with adverse cardiovascular outcomes [3–5]. This relationship is independent of systolic blood pressure and occurs in a temporal sequence consistent with a causal relationship [6]. The European Society of Cardiology and European Society of Hypertension guidelines published in 2007 indicate that an accelerated heart rate should be considered an independent risk factor and potential target for pharmacotherapy particularly in high-risk patients [7].

It is probably not surprising that the number of cardiovascular events (although not mortality) increased in the sibutramine-treated patients in the Sibutramine Cardiovascular Outcomes (SCOUT) trial [8]. Indeed it is possible that the SCOUT may have underestimated risk of sibutramine. The initial open-label phase allowed the exclusion of those particularly sensitive to the hypertensive effects or increased heart rate induced by sibutramine [8]. On the other hand, a subgroup of patients appears to benefit. Subsequent analyses of the SCOUT data have shown that a modest weight loss (~3 kg) achieved in the lead-in period appeared to offset the increased event rate, and weight loss of 3–10 kg at 6–12 months was associated with a reduced cardiovascular event rate in those with severe, moderate, or mild cardiovascular disease [9]. An analysis of heart rate change in relation to weight loss and cardiovascular outcomes would be of considerable interest, along with an analysis of effect modification in relation to concomitant medications; a particularly large number of participants in the high-risk group were taking beta-blockers. Further, in a recent study, despite significant weight loss in sibutramine-treated diabetics, leptin, TNF-alpha, adiponectin, and hs-CRP did not decrease in comparison to the control group [10].

Rimonabant

Rimonabant lowers both systolic and diastolic blood pressure and triglycerides. Beneficial effects on HDL glucose and HbA1c reported in early reviews [1, 11] were not found to be significant compared to placebo in a recent systemic review and meta-analysis [12]. This is consistent with recent experimental data showing that improvements in insulin regulation of free fatty acid and glucose metabolism with rimonabant treatment in humans are no greater than that predicted by weight loss alone [13].

Psychiatric side effects, in particular anxiety and depression, were frequently associated with rimonabant use [14], and, although relatively rare, the significant risk of suicidality and lack of data on the any health-related quality of life benefits ultimately resulted in the withdrawal of the drug from all markets worldwide.

The effect of rimonabant on incident cardiovascular events and type 2 diabetes mellitus as well as mortality remains unknown; a 5 % loss of body weight over a 30-month period with rimonabant was insufficient to modify atherosclerosis progression in the carotid artery in obese patients with metabolic syndrome [15]. Potential benefits for specific obesity-related complications – for example, the demonstration of weight-independent effects to reduce liver insulin resistance [16] and ameliorate fatty liver [17, 18] – were at a relatively early stages of exploration. A very small study, largely as a consequence of being prematurely terminated by the withdrawal of rimonabant worldwide, suggested a potential psychiatric benefit for people with schizophrenia or schizoaffective disorder taking second-generation antipsychotics [19]. The serotonergic system appears to be the most likely candidate mediating the psychiatric side effects of CB1 receptor antagonists [20], suggesting the potential for treatment with SSRIs.

In addition, polymorphisms of the CB1 receptor gene (CNR1) alone or together with the gene of the serotonin transporter (SLC6A4) may identify individuals at high or low risk, therefore facilitating a personalized approach to drug selection [20].

Clinical Trials Verse the Real World

Patterns of pharmacotherapy use in the community are of interest and informative, particularly since the population of users may not reflect those enrolled in the trials. In the USA, for example, among insured patients, use decreased from 1 % in 2002 to 0.7 % in 2005 (most notably for sibutramine and orlistat), and of these only 11–18 % continued to use them for longer than 3 months. More than half (57 %) of the antiobesity medication users were concurrently taking narcotics and 38 % antidepressants [21]. The majority of UK adolescents prescribed sibutramine, rimonabant, or orlistat off-license discontinue the drugs before weight benefit, suggesting they are poorly tolerated or poorly efficacious when used in the general population [22].

In the context of clinical trials, depressive symptoms at baseline were a significant predictor of both attrition and weight-loss success, and non-completion of the trial was significantly less likely when early weight loss occurred [23].

Obesity is not a homogeneous condition. Moreover, affected individuals have a range of physical and psychological comorbidities of varying degrees of severity and concomitant medication use that may coexist with variable behavioral, environmental, and psychosocial factors. Clinical trials enroll a select subset of patients, which may not reflect the broader use once marketed nor identify those most likely to benefit.

Whether any reduction in energy intake, without optimizing the overall macronutrient and micronutrient content of the diet, may limit any long-term benefit also remains to be answered.

The side-effect profile, questionable benefits, and long-term risks in a significant number of individuals should have argued strongly against a strategy to promote widespread use of these medications. But there are undoubtedly particular groups of individuals with either specific or combinations of comorbidities that benefit from one or another of these drugs either in terms of magnitude of weight loss, amelioration of comorbidities, or both. That potential is now denied. And governments, now more than ever, will reasonably ask the question whether expenditure on pharmacotherapy of this sort is a better investment than alternative cardiovascular risk reduction strategies, both pharmacological and non-pharmacological.

What Lessons Might We Learn?

The problem is not necessarily the drugs themselves; rather it is the push for rapid development to market and the regulatory environment (limited patents) that drives this. The intention is high-volume sales, with strategies to accomplish this being determined by business development and marketing priorities, rather than being informed by careful clinical research, analysis, and prudent decision-making. Scientific advisory boards should not just be used as marketing tools without serious intent to garner and follow reasoned expert advice.

Because many outcomes are not assessed in clinical trials, and participants may not be forthcoming with the information, significant side effects may not be detected. Examples include erectile dysfunction in men and lower urinary tract symptoms in both sexes. Trials should be designed that reflect use in the real world, and regulatory approval should not be provided in their absence. The exclusion of particular patient groups means a benefit may be lost – for example, rimonabant in patients taking SSRIs. Strategies to mitigate adverse effects – for example, the prescription of an SSRI for emergent neuropsychiatric symptoms or even a trial of combination therapy – may have produced a beneficial outcome.

Drugs should be launched with more sophisticated labeling and protocols for use initially among specialist groups, with careful monitoring by the use of registries and then wider use permitted in accordance with the benefits demonstrated to occur. In turn, governments/regulators need to substantially prolong patent protection to make this approach worthwhile.

References

1. Rucker D, Padwal R, Li SK, Curioni C, Lau DC. Long term pharmacotherapy for obesity and overweight: updated meta-analysis. BMJ. 2007;335(7631):1194–9.
2. Johansson K, Sundstrom J, Neovius K, Rossner S, Neovius M. Long-term changes in blood pressure following orlistat and sibutramine treatment: a meta-analysis. Obes Rev. 2010;11(11):777–91.
3. Greenland P, Daviglus ML, Dyer AR, Liu K, Huang CF, Goldberger JJ, et al. Resting heart rate is a risk factor for cardiovascular and noncardiovascular mortality: the Chicago Heart Association Detection Project in Industry. Am J Epidemiol. 1999;149(9):853–62.
4. Palatini P, Casiglia E, Julius S, Pessina AC. High heart rate: a risk factor for cardiovascular death in elderly men. Arch Intern Med. 1999;159(6):585–92.
5. Miot A, Ragot S, Hammi W, Saulnier PJ, Sosner P, Piguel X, et al. Prognostic value of resting heart rate on cardiovascular and renal outcomes in type 2 diabetic patients: a competing risk analysis in a prospective cohort. Diabetes Care. 2012;35(10):2069–75.
6. Cooney MT, Vartiainen E, Laatikainen T, Juolevi A, Dudina A, Graham IM. Elevated resting heart rate is an independent risk factor for cardiovascular disease in healthy men and women. Am Heart J. 2010;159(4):612–9.e3.
7. Mancia G, De Backer G, Dominiczak A, Cifkova R, Fagard R, Germano G, et al. 2007 ESH-ESC practice guidelines for the management of arterial hypertension: ESH-ESC task force on the management of arterial hypertension. J Hypertens. 2007;25(9):1751–62.
8. James WP, Caterson ID, Coutinho W, Finer N, Van Gaal LF, Maggioni AP, et al. Effect of sibutramine on cardiovascular outcomes in overweight and obese subjects. N Engl J Med. 2010;363(10):905–17.
9. Caterson ID, Finer N, Coutinho W, Van Gaal LF, Maggioni AP, Torp-Pedersen C, et al. Maintained intentional weight loss reduces cardiovascular outcomes: results from the Sibutramine Cardiovascular OUTcomes (SCOUT) trial. Diabetes Obes Metab. 2012;14(6):523–30.
10. Derosa G, Maffioli P, Ferrari I, Palumbo I, Randazzo S, D'Angelo A, et al. Variation of inflammatory parameters after sibutramine treatment compared to placebo in type 2 diabetic patients. J Clin Pharm Ther. 2011;36(5):592–601.
11. Burch J, McKenna C, Palmer S, Norman G, Glanville J, Sculpher M, et al. Rimonabant for the treatment of overweight and obese people. Health Technol Assess. 2009;13 Suppl 3:13–22.

12. Zhou YH, Ma XQ, Wu C, Lu J, Zhang SS, Guo J, et al. Effect of anti-obesity drug on cardiovascular risk factors: a systematic review and meta-analysis of randomized controlled trials. PLoS One. 2012;7(6):e39062.

13. Triay J, Mundi M, Klein S, Toledo FG, Smith SR, Abu-Lebdeh H, et al. Does rimonabant independently affect free fatty acid and glucose metabolism? J Clin Endocrinol Metabol. 2012;97(3):819–27.

14. Nathan PJ, O'Neill BV, Napolitano A, Bullmore ET. Neuropsychiatric adverse effects of centrally acting antiobesity drugs. CNS Neurosci Ther. 2011;17(5):490–505.

15. O'Leary DH, Reuwer AQ, Nissen SE, Despres JP, Deanfield JE, Brown MW, et al. Effect of rimonabant on carotid intima-media thickness (CIMT) progression in patients with abdominal obesity and metabolic syndrome: the AUDITOR Trial. Heart. 2011;97(14):1143–50.

16. Kim SP, Woolcott OO, Hsu IR, Stefanoski D, Harrison LN, Zheng D, et al. CB(1) antagonism restores hepatic insulin sensitivity without normalization of adiposity in diet-induced obese dogs. Am J Physiol Endocrinol Metab. 2012;302(10):E1261–8.

17. Banasch M, Goetze O, Schmidt WE, Meier JJ. Rimonabant as a novel therapeutic option for nonalcoholic steatohepatitis. Liver Int. 2007;27(8):1152–5.

18. Wierzbicki AS, Pendleton S, McMahon Z, Dar A, Oben J, Crook MA, et al. Rimonabant improves cholesterol, insulin resistance and markers of non-alcoholic fatty liver in morbidly obese patients: a retrospective cohort study. Int J Clin Pract. 2011;65(6):713–5.

19. Kelly DL, Gorelick DA, Conley RR, Boggs DL, Linthicum J, Liu F, et al. Effects of the cannabinoid-1 receptor antagonist rimonabant on psychiatric symptoms in overweight people with schizophrenia: a randomized, double-blind, pilot study. J Clin Psychopharmacol. 2011;31(1):86–91.

20. Lazary J, Juhasz G, Hunyady L, Bagdy G. Personalized medicine can pave the way for the safe use of CB(1) receptor antagonists. Trends Pharmacol Sci. 2011;32(5):270–80.

21. Bolen SD, Clark JM, Richards TM, Shore AD, Goodwin SM, Weiner JP. Trends in and patterns of obesity reduction medication use in an insured cohort. Obesity. 2010;18(1):206–9.

22. Viner RM, Hsia Y, Neubert A, Wong IC. Rise in antiobesity drug prescribing for children and adolescents in the UK: a population-based study. Br J Clin Pharmacol. 2009;68(6):844–51.

23. Fabricatore AN, Wadden TA, Moore RH, Butryn ML, Heymsfield SB, Nguyen AM. Predictors of attrition and weight loss success: results from a randomized controlled trial. Behav Res Ther. 2009;47(8):685–91.

Chapter 29
Laparoscopic Adjustable Gastric Banding: The Physician's Choice in Bariatric Surgery

John B. Dixon

The laparoscopic adjustable gastric banding (LAGB) procedure is one of the most remarkable advances in weight management. The clear need to adjust the gastric "restriction" component of bariatric surgery to achieve great results was seen independently by two of the greatest innovators in bariatric surgery [1, 2]. The simultaneous light bulb moments, with clever modification, were soon adapted for the emerging laparoscopic era of surgery and were the very first laparoscopic bariatric procedures. Ongoing improvements in band technology, placement, and management have reduced morbidity and long-term complications and improved the effectiveness of LAGB. Today, LAGB offers patients fewer procedural complications and decreased hospital time compared with other weight-loss surgeries [3, 4] and excellent sustained weight loss if managed appropriately.

J.B. Dixon, MBBS, PhD, FRACGP, FRCPEdin, NHMRC
Primary Care Research Unit, Clinical Obesity Research,
and Weight Assessment and Management Clinic,
Baker IDI Heart and Diabetes Institute, Monash University,
75 Commercial Road, Melbourne, VIC 3004, Australia
e-mail: john.dixon@bakeridi.edu.au

D.W. Haslam et al. (eds.), *Controversies in Obesity*,
DOI 10.1007/978-1-4471-2834-2_29,
© Springer-Verlag London 2014

A better understanding of the mechanism of action of the band and other bariatric surgeries is emerging, but no bariatric surgical procedure is "restrictive," absolutely limiting intake, and none significantly delay the transit or absorption of food. If they did, then reducing meal size would simply be followed by more frequent meals. We have clearly shown through a double-blinded crossover trial that a well-adjusted band produced earlier satiation and excellent prolonged satiety following a small test meal [5]. The mechanism of action is via a rich plexus of gastric wall stretch receptors and vagal afferents situated immediately below the gastroesophageal junction and in a rodent model; the effect of the band can be switched on and off with adjustment and abolished by afferent nerve blockade [6]. In managing patients following LAGB surgery, it is critical that the whole practice team and each patient understand how the band works.

The LAGB procedure has the broadest range of indications of any bariatric surgery today. The most commonly used band, the Lap-Band, is now FDA approved for use in the BMI range of 30–35 with comorbidity. Not only does the band have the best early safety profile, it has ideal attributes for those wanting to achieve healthy sustained weight loss. The weight loss is gentle and progressive, allowing adequate adaptation and optimal nutrition to best preserve muscle mass during weight loss. This procedure allows a greater proportion of fat to be lost and fat-free tissues to be retained [7]. There is no GI diversion or resection involved such that micronutrient deficiencies, which predictably occur with more disruptive procedures, are not experienced. The controlled effect on weight loss is optimal for younger patients who are yet to maximize bone mass; for women planning a family, where balanced nutrition and appropriate weight change during pregnancy is important for mother and child; in the elderly, in whom weight loss should be controlled and must be accompanied by excellent nutrition, preservation of muscle, bone, and physical function; and in those with complex serious comorbidity where a safe gentle procedure followed by controlled sustained weight loss with excellent nutrition is required to optimize function and health outcomes.

LAGB surgery is the most standardized and reproducible bariatric surgery performed today. Weight loss is progressive over 2 or even 3 years and then appears sustainable. At 5 years postsurgery, mean percentage excess weight loss (% EWL) is 50–55 %, or 20–25 % of total weight. LAGB surgery also has the most rigorous evidence base, with years of audited studies prior to US FDA approval and series of randomized controlled trials showing it to be consistently superior to medical weight-loss therapies [8–11]. There is no better treatment for obesity-related comorbidity than sustained weight loss, and weight loss following LAGB surgery is accompanied by improvements in, or normalization of, insulin sensitivity and glycemia, obesity-related dyslipidemia, C-reactive protein (CRP), and other pro-inflammatory cytokine levels, nonalcoholic fatty liver disease, sleep disturbances including obstructive sleep apnea and daytime sleepiness, and ovulatory function and fertility in women with polycystic ovary syndrome [12, 13]. Perhaps the most important outcomes from a patient's perspective include enhanced quality of life, body image [14], and fewer symptoms of depression [15]. The other compelling health outcome following LAGB includes reduced mortality compared with obese community controls [16, 17]. LAGB however, appears consistently to be more cost-effective than RYGB [18] and even presents the rare scenario in health of a return on investment [19].

The reversible less-disruptive nature of LAGB lends itself to low procedural risks, shorter operations [20], and surgeries performed in day-stay ambulatory surgical centers [21, 22]. The incidence of late complications has varied, but there are clear indications that improved placement and management techniques have reduced incidence. Looking at cohorts of greater than 500 patients at baseline and followed at least 2 years has shown a 5 % reoperation rate for proximal pouch enlargement [23]. Erosion or migration of the band into the lumen of the stomach has an incidence of 1.5 % as reported in a recent meta-analysis of almost 16,000 patients, with lower rates being found with increased surgical experience [24]. Higher revision and explants rates were described in early series before band placement and adjustment techniques had been refined [25, 26].

Bariatric surgery is not a stand-alone quick-fix solution; rather, it is a tool that is integrated with the chronic disease management of serious complex obesity. Bariatric surgery aftercare, therefore, does not sit well with a surgical care model. As for all chronic disease management, bariatric surgery requires indefinite follow-up, with access to a multidisciplinary integrated team to optimize health outcomes and minimize the risks and complications. Physicians are ideally placed to manage this ongoing care of patients, and the LAGB specifically is a physician's choice of bariatric procedure, due to its adjustability, which allows for the changing needs of a patient over time, similar to a cardiac pacemaker.

With the success of a patient-orientated, physician practice-led integrated model of chronic disease care [27, 28], rather than a surgical model of care, the LAGB has the ability to be among the most safe, effective, and accessible treatments for severe chronic obesity.

Disclosures   Associate Professor Dixon is a consultant for Allergan Inc., Metagenics Inc. (Bariatric Advantage), and formerly Scientific Intake. He is also on the medical advisory board for Optifast, Nestle Australia. Our laboratory currently receives research funding from Medtronics Inc. (formally Ardian Inc.), Abbott (formerly Solvay) Pharmaceuticals, Allergan Inc., Servier and Scientific Intake. These organizations played no role in the design, analysis, or interpretation of data described here nor preparation, review, or approval of the manuscript.

References

1. Hallberg D. Why the operation I prefer is adjustable gastric banding. Obes Surg. 1991;1:187–8.
2. Kuzmak LI, Yap IS, McGuire L, Dixon JS, Young MP. Surgery for morbid obesity. Using an inflatable gastric band. AORN J. 1990;51:1307–24.
3. Flum DR, Belle SH, King WC, Wahed AS, Berk P, Chapman W, et al. Perioperative safety in the longitudinal assessment of bariatric surgery. N Engl J Med. 2009;361:445–54.
4. DeMaria EJ, Pate V, Warthen M, Winegar DA. Baseline data from American society for metabolic and bariatric surgery-designated

bariatric surgery centers of excellence using the bariatric outcomes longitudinal database. Surg Obes Relat Dis. 2010;6:347–55.

5. Dixon AF, Dixon JB, O'Brien PE. Laparoscopic adjustable gastric banding induces prolonged satiety: a randomized blind crossover study. J Clin Endocrinol Metab. 2005;90:813–9.

6. Kampe J, Stefanidis A, Lockie SH, Brown WA, Dixon JB, Odoi A, et al. Neural and humoral changes associated with the adjustable gastric band: Insights from a rodent model. Int J Obes (Lond). 2012;36:1403–11.

7. Chaston TB, Dixon JB, O'Brien PE. Changes in fat-free mass during significant weight loss: a systematic review. Int J Obes (Lond). 2007; 31:743–50.

8. O'Brien PE, Dixon JB, Laurie C, Skinner S, Proietto J, McNeil J, et al. Treatment of mild to moderate obesity with laparoscopic adjustable gastric banding or an intensive medical program: a randomized trial. Ann Intern Med. 2006;144:625–33.

9. O'Brien PE, Sawyer SM, Laurie C, Brown WA, Skinner S, Veit F, et al. Laparoscopic adjustable gastric banding in severely obese adolescents: a randomized trial. JAMA. 2010;303:519–26.

10. Dixon JB, O'Brien PE, Playfair J, Chapman L, Schachter LM, Skinner S, et al. Adjustable gastric banding and conventional therapy for type 2 diabetes: a randomized controlled trial. JAMA. 2008;299:316–23.

11. Dixon JB, Schachter LM, O'Brien PE, Jones K, Grima M, Lambert G, et al. Surgical vs conventional therapy for weight loss treatment of obstructive sleep apnea: a randomized controlled trial. JAMA. 2012;308:1142–9.

12. Dixon JB, O'Brien PE. Changes in comorbidities and improvements in quality of life after lap-band placement. Am J Surg. 2002;184:S51–4.

13. Chen SB, Lee YC, Ser KH, Chen JC, Chen SC, Hsieh HF, et al. Serum c-reactive protein and white blood cell count in morbidly obese surgical patients. Obes Surg. 2009;19:461–6.

14. Dixon JB, Dixon ME, O'Brien PE. Body image: appearance orientation and evaluation in the severely obese. Changes with weight loss. Obes Surg. 2002;12:65–71.

15. Dixon JB, Dixon ME, O'Brien PE. Depression in association with severe obesity: changes with weight loss. Arch Intern Med. 2003;163:2058–65.

16. Peeters A, O'Brien PE, Laurie C, Anderson M, Wolfe R, Flum D, et al. Substantial intentional weight loss and mortality in the severely obese. Ann Surg. 2007;246:1028–33.

17. Busetto L, Mirabelli D, Petroni ML, Mazza M, Favretti F, Segato G, et al. Comparative long-term mortality after laparoscopic adjustable gastric banding versus nonsurgical controls. Surg Obes Relat Dis. 2007;3:496–502; discussion 502.

18. Salem L, Devlin A, Sullivan SD, Flum DR. Cost-effectiveness analysis of laparoscopic gastric bypass, adjustable gastric banding, and nonoperative weight loss interventions. Surg Obes Relat Dis. 2008;4:26–32.

19. Finkelstein EA, Brown DS. Return on investment for bariatric surgery. Am J Manag Care. 2008;14:561–2.

20. Jan JC, Hong D, Bardaro SJ, July LV, Patterson EJ. Comparative study between laparoscopic adjustable gastric banding and laparoscopic gastric bypass: single-institution, 5-year experience in bariatric surgery. Surg Obes Relat Dis. 2007;3:42–50; discussion 50–1.
21. Watkins BM, Ahroni JH, Michaelson R, Montgomery KF, Abrams RE, Erlitz MD, et al. Laparoscopic adjustable gastric banding in an ambulatory surgery center. Surg Obes Relat Dis. 2008;4:S56–62.
22. Cobourn C, Mumford D, Chapman MA, Wells L. Laparoscopic gastric banding is safe in outpatient surgical centers. Obes Surg. 2010;20:415–22.
23. Singhal R, Bryant C, Kitchen M, Khan KS, Deeks J, Guo B, Super P. Band slippage and erosion after laparoscopic gastric banding: a meta-analysis. Surg Endosc. 2010;24:2980–6.
24. Egberts K, Brown WA, O'Brien PE. Systematic review of erosion after laparoscopic adjustable gastric banding. Obes Surg. 2011;21:1272–9.
25. Westling A, Bjurling K, Ohrvall M, Gustavsson S. Silicone-adjustable gastric banding: disappointing results. Obes Surg. 1998;8:467–74.
26. DeMaria EJ, Sugerman HJ, Meador JG, Doty JM, Kellum JM, Wolfe L, et al. High failure rate after laparoscopic adjustable silicone gastric banding for treatment of morbid obesity. Ann Surg. 2001;233:809–18.
27. Wagner EH, Davis C, Schaefer J, Von Korff M, Austin B. A survey of leading chronic disease management programs: are they consistent with the literature? Manag Care Q. 1999;7:56–66.
28. Gregg EW, Cheng YJ, Saydah S, Cowie C, Garfield S, Geiss L, et al. Trends in death rates among U.S. Adults with and without diabetes between 1997 and 2006: findings from the national health interview survey. Diabetes Care. 2012;35:1252–7.

Chapter 30
Challenges Faced by the Bariatric Multidisciplinary Team

Wen Bun Leong and Shahrad Taheri

The prevalence of obesity is rising alarmingly worldwide [1]. Obesity is associated with a multitude of chronic disorders resulting in major economic and social challenges. Obesity and associated disorders are likely to result in great pressures on health-care systems. Therapies for obesity included lifestyle interventions, pharmacological treatment, and bariatric surgery. Dietary and lifestyle modifications have been shown to result in modest weight reduction [2, 3]. Currently in the UK, orlistat, a lipase inhibitor, is the only drug licensed for obesity treatment with limited success in weight loss. Hopefully, emerging pharmacological agents will increasingly allow safe and effective management of obesity. To date,

W.B. Leong, MBChB(Hons), MRCP
Diabetes and Endocrinology, Birmingham Heartlands Hospital,
Heart of England NHS Foundation Trust, Bordesley Green East,
Birmingham, West Midlands B9 5SS, UK
e-mail: w.leong@bham.ac.uk

S. Taheri, BSc, MSc, MBBS, PhD, FRCP (✉)
Department of Medicine,
Weill Cornell Medical College - Qatar,
Qatar Foundation - Education City, 24144, Qatar
e-mail: staheri@me.com

D.W. Haslam et al. (eds.), *Controversies in Obesity*,
DOI 10.1007/978-1-4471-2834-2_30,
© Springer-Verlag London 2014

bariatric surgery is the most effective treatment for extreme obesity, especially when complicated by comorbidities such as diabetes [4]. The most common bariatric procedures performed are laparoscopic Roux-en-Y gastric bypass surgery (LRYGB), laparoscopic adjustable gastric band (LAGB), and laparoscopic sleeve gastrectomy (LSG).

Although bariatric surgery is very effective in weight management, it also carries risks and harms [5–7]. Therefore, patients who are seeking bariatric surgery require assessment by a multidisciplinary team (MDT). An MDT consists of a group of health-care professionals "with various expertise, responsible for individual decisions, who hold a common purpose and meet together to communicate, share, and consolidate knowledge from which plans are made" [8].

A physician specializing in obesity, or a bariatric physician, usually leads the MDT; his role includes assessing and excluding medical causes of obesity; performing investigations; devising, implementing, and monitoring treatment plans for obesity-related diseases [9]; management of nutritional deficiencies for patients post bariatric surgery [9, 10]; and finally, maintaining good communication with the primary care team and other health-care professionals. The physician specializing in obesity should also provide good leadership to the team. A list of the MDT members and roles is shown in Table 30.1.

The MDT should meet at regular intervals with frequency depending on patient volume, usually weekly at a center of excellence. Different members of the MDT can chair the meeting. Various treatment options will be explored during the meeting, leading to a more structured, standardized, and coordinated patient management plan. It also provides better and more effective information sharing between health-care professionals and may serve as opportunities for the professional development and training of team members as well as trainees [11, 12]. Finally, the MDT may also function as a portal for the identification of potential patients for research and clinical trials [13]. A standardized pro forma for each patient is useful during MDT meetings, and data can be collected for future audit of the meetings as well as decisions.

TABLE 30.1 A list of bariatric multidisciplinary team (MDT) members

Team members	Roles
Physician specializing in obesity (bariatric physician)	Team leader
	Assess medical causes of obesity
	Manage obesity-related medical diseases
	Monitor and implements weight-management programs
	Manage nutritional deficiencies post bariatric surgery
	Communicate to primary care team and other specialists
	Patient advocacy and support
	Audit, service evaluation, and research
	Education and training
Bariatric surgeon	Assess suitability for bariatric surgery
	Provide impartial information on surgical procedures to patients
	Informed consent for bariatric surgery
	Devise a postoperative follow-up schedule with the MDT
	Patient advocacy and support
	Audit, service evaluation, and research
	Education and training
Specialist weight-management dietitian	First portal of contact for patients in most centers
	Explain and implement suitable dietetic regime to individual patients
	Assess for any significant eating disorders
	Provide dietetic information for patients prior and after bariatric surgery
	Patient advocacy and support
	Audit, service evaluation, and research
	Education and training

(continued)

TABLE 30.1 (continued)

Team members	Roles
Clinical bariatric nurse specialist	Contribute to medical assessments
	Help prepare and monitor patients perioperatively
	Provide clinical and psychological support to patients
	Promote collaboration between team members
	Help in administration and scoring of questionnaires
	Bariatric nursing education to different departments in hospital
	Can act as bariatric coordinator
	Patient advocacy and support
	Audit, service evaluation, and research
	Assist in enrolment of patients in research studies
	Education and training
Psychologist/ psychiatrist	Assess any major mental health issues, e.g., depression
	Assess and manage eating disorders
	Patient advocacy and support
	Audit, service evaluation, and research
	Education and training
Bariatric coordinator	Monitor and facilitate transition of patients into various clinics
	Organize MDT meetings
Administration staff	Ensure smooth running of clinics
	First point of contact for primary care team
	May involve in data collection for future audits/database

Challenges can occur in the setup as well as running of an MDT. Cost is one factor, and gathering health-care professionals with various expertise to meet together (MDT meeting) at a specific time in a specific place can be difficult. Also, decisions made by the MDT may lack input from patients and may cause reduction in patient satisfaction. Thus, it is important that the MDT member with the greatest knowledge and contact with the patient should lead the discussion, providing a good understanding of the patient and their needs and wishes. Conflicts can occur within the team; this could be due to several factors, including lack of clarity of team member roles, lack of interaction between team members, and miscommunications with patients [14, 15]. Patient information leaflets or brochures as well as writing and posting clinical letters to patients could help reduce patient miscommunication and misinformation.

Due to the globalization of health care, individuals may seek to have bariatric surgery in a place other than their country of origin. In short, medical tourism is gradually on the rise. Reasons for medical tourism include inaccessible service or care in one's own country of residence, long waiting lists, high cost, or patients' perception that they will receive better care or outcomes [16]. Unfortunately, complications and, in some instances, death may occur when patients return home or an inadequate support and follow-up plan is implemented [16, 17]. In other cases, patients might not receive structured workup prior to surgery, which may affect their peri- and postoperative outcomes [16]. These individuals will subsequently present to the local specialist weight-management services with various presentations and possible complications from the procedures such as atypical infections. These cases are often complex and pose one of the challenges for the MDT as well as additional economic costs to the local health-care system. The MDT may need to provide medicolegal input in some case, requiring additional training. A bariatric center in Canada reported CDN$162,791 additional cost from medical tourism [16]. The full impact of medical tourism for bariatric surgery towards the NHS has been little studied.

Apart from medical tourism, the specialist weight-management services team may also need to manage patients who have sought treatment in private centers within their country of origin. The care and outcomes from private centers will depend on many factors, such as the level of accreditation and inspection of medical facilities by regulatory bodies, regulation of the competency of the health-care professionals, as well as standard of practice [17]. In some instances, complications still arise and patients may present to their local hospital specialist weight-management services team for further management. These problems can be circumvented by appropriate designation of all centers for provision of specialist weight management and bariatric surgery, whether public or private.

Obesity is a chronic condition and should be managed by an MDT with various expertise that can ensure good short- and long-term patient outcomes. Although not systematically studied, the advantages of the MDT approach are undeniable. However, barriers and challenges are also present. These can be overcome through pathway development, definition of roles, sharing information, and good communication. Finally, with the gradual rise in private practices, locally as well as internationally, the MDT should be prepared to manage more complex cases.

Declaration of Interests   Dr. Wen Leong is funded through an unrestricted educational grant from Allergan. Dr Shahrad Taheri is funded by the National Institute for Health Research (NIHR) through the Collaborations for Leadership in Applied Health Research and Care for Birmingham and Black Country (CLAHRC-BBC) program. The views expressed in this publication are not necessarily those of the NIHR, the Department of Health, NHS South Birmingham, University of Birmingham, or the CLAHRC-BBC Theme 8 Management/Steering Group.

Dr. Shahrad Taheri has received educational funding support from Lilly UK. He has received research support from Novo Nordisk, Philips Respironics, and Resmed.

References

1. Wang YC, McPherson K, Marsh T, Gortmaker SL, Brown M. Health and economic burden of the projected obesity trends in the USA and the UK. Lancet. 2011;378(9793):815–25. Epub 2011/08/30.

2. Tuomilehto J, Lindstrom J, Eriksson JG, Valle TT, Hamalainen H, Ilanne-Parikka P, et al. Prevention of type 2 diabetes mellitus by changes in lifestyle among subjects with impaired glucose tolerance. N Engl J Med. 2001;344(18):1343–50. Epub 2001/05/03.

3. Knowler WC, Barrett-Connor E, Fowler SE, Hamman RF, Lachin JM, Walker EA, et al. Reduction in the incidence of type 2 diabetes with lifestyle intervention or metformin. N Engl J Med. 2002;346(6):393–403. Epub 2002/02/08.

4. Buchwald H, Avidor Y, Braunwald E, Jensen MD, Pories W, Fahrbach K, et al. Bariatric surgery: a systematic review and meta-analysis. JAMA. 2004;292(14):1724–37. Epub 2004/10/14.

5. Buchwald H, Estok R, Fahrbach K, Banel D, Sledge I. Trends in mortality in bariatric surgery: a systematic review and meta-analysis. Surgery. 2007;142(4):621–32; discussion 32–5. Epub 2007/10/24.

6. Demaria EJ, Winegar DA, Pate VW, Hutcher NE, Ponce J, Pories WJ. Early postoperative outcomes of metabolic surgery to treat diabetes from sites participating in the ASMBS bariatric surgery center of excellence program as reported in the Bariatric Outcomes Longitudinal Database. Ann Surg. 2010;252(3):559–66; discussion 66–7. Epub 2010/08/27.

7. Flum DR, Belle SH, King WC, Wahed AS, Berk P, Chapman W, et al. Perioperative safety in the longitudinal assessment of bariatric surgery. N Engl J Med. 2009;361(5):445–54. Epub 2009/07/31.

8. Tremblay D, Roberge D, Cazale L, Touati N, Maunsell E, Latreille J, et al. Evaluation of the impact of interdisciplinarity in cancer care. BMC Health Serv Res. 2011;11:144. Epub 2011/06/07.

9. Saltzman E, Anderson W, Apovian CM, Boulton H, Chamberlain A, Cullum-Dugan D, et al. Criteria for patient selection and multidisciplinary evaluation and treatment of the weight loss surgery patient. Obes Res. 2005;13(2):234–43. Epub 2005/04/01.

10. Mechanick JI, Kushner RF, Sugerman HJ, Gonzalez-Campoy JM, Collazo-Clavell ML, Spitz AF, et al. American Association of Clinical Endocrinologists, The Obesity Society, and American Society for Metabolic & Bariatric Surgery medical guidelines for clinical practice for the perioperative nutritional, metabolic, and nonsurgical support of the bariatric surgery patient. Obesity (Silver Spring). 2009;17 Suppl 1:S1–70, v. Epub 2009/05/16.

11. Bakemeier RF, Beck S, Murphy JR. Educational and consultative functions, topics, and methods of hospital general tumor conferences. J Cancer Educ. 1995;9(4):217–25. Epub 1995/01/01.

12. Sarff M, Rogers W, Blanke C, Vetto JT. Evaluation of the tumor board as a Continuing Medical Education (CME) activity: is it useful? J Cancer Educ. 2008;23(1):51–6. Epub 2008/04/30.

13. Kuroki L, Stuckey A, Hirway P, Raker CA, Bandera CA, DiSilvestro PA, et al. Addressing clinical trials: can the multidisciplinary Tumor Board improve participation? A study from an academic women's cancer program. Gynecol Oncol. 2010;116(3):295–300. Epub 2010/01/01.

14. Jenkins VA, Fallowfield LJ, Poole K. Are members of multidisciplinary teams in breast cancer aware of each other's informational roles? Qual Health Care. 2001;10(2):70–5. Epub 2001/06/05.
15. Catt S, Fallowfield L, Jenkins V, Langridge C, Cox A. The informational roles and psychological health of members of 10 oncology multidisciplinary teams in the UK. Br J Cancer. 2005;93(10):1092–7. Epub 2005/10/20.
16. Birch DW, Vu L, Karmali S, Stoklossa CJ, Sharma AM. Medical tourism in bariatric surgery. Am J Surg. 2010;199(5):604–8. Epub 2010/03/30.
17. Turner L. News media reports of patient deaths following 'medical tourism' for cosmetic surgery and bariatric surgery. Dev World Bioeth. 2012;12(1):21–34. Epub 2012/03/17.

Chapter 31
The Controversies Around Roux-en-Y Gastric Bypass

Carel W. le Roux

Background

Roux-en-Y gastric bypass (RYGB) surgery is more effective than nonsurgical treatments of obesity to sustain long-term weight loss [1]. During the RYGB procedure, the stomach is divided into an upper gastric pouch, which is 15–30 mL in volume, and a lower gastric remnant. The gastric pouch is anastomosed to the jejunum after it has been divided some 30–75 cm distal to the ligament of Treitz; this distal part is brought up as a "Roux limb." The excluded biliary limb, including the gastric remnant, is connected to the bowel 75–150 cm distal to the gastrojejunostomy.

The outcomes following RYGB vary between patients, and predicting individual outcomes is difficult. Below each outcome is reviewed individually and the controversies that surround it are discussed.

C.W. le Roux, MBChB, MSc, FRCP, FRCPath, PhD
Department of Pathology,
Diabetes Complications Research Centre,
Conway Institute, University College Dublin,
Dublin, Ireland
e-mail: carel.leroux@ucd.ie

D.W. Haslam et al. (eds.), *Controversies in Obesity*,
DOI 10.1007/978-1-4471-2834-2_31,
© Springer-Verlag London 2014

Airway

RYGB is associated with impressive remission rates for obstructive sleep apnea (OSA) in prospective cohort studies. However, randomized controlled studies are lacking, and where such studies have been done with gastric banding, only the severity of OSA is improved and full remission is not more frequent than nonsurgical weight loss [2].

Body Weight

RYGB results on average in 25 % long-term loss maintenance, but weight regain can be a problem in a substantial number of patients [1]. The mechanisms for weight loss are controversial: dogmatic restriction and calorie malabsorption were proposed as explanations, but these have been discredited through careful biological measurements [3]. It is now accepted that neurohormonal signals from the gut to the brain attenuate appetite [4], but although several animal studies also suggest a shift in food preference to lower fat and lower glycemic index carbohydrates, the prospective human studies with sufficiently robust methodologies are still awaited [5]. Enhanced energy expenditure after RYGB has also raised controversy; it now appears that although basal metabolic rate may be reduced after RYGB, the postprandial thermogenesis is sufficiently raised to result in an overall increase in 24-h energy expenditure [6].

Cardiovascular Disease

Carefully conducted long-term cohort studies show reduced cardiovascular mortality and morbidity after RYGB [1]. The mechanism is unclear, but improvements in glucose metabolism, blood lipid profiles, and hypertension probably contribute. Only raised fasting insulin levels and not BMI predict which patients benefit, suggesting that obese patients without insulin resistance should not be encouraged to have RYGB based on a perceived mortality benefit. Moreover, the lack of randomized controlled trials makes such claims even for those with type 2 diabetes questionable. Combination of statins, metformin, and angiotensin-converting enzyme inhibitors has reduced death significantly in nonsurgical patients, and this makes powering a future RCT very difficult due to the low absolute incidence of cardiovascular events in patients prior to RYGB.

Diabetes

Approximately 25 % of patients undergoing RYGB have type 2 diabetes (T2DM), and often, the aim is to cure them. The American Diabetes Association criteria defining "cure of diabetes" are now more stringent, and there are no RCT data to compare cure between RYGB and nonsurgical care, because to define cure, 5 years must elapse after the RYGB [7]. The best RCT data available suggest 41 % remission rate at 1 year after RYGB, but a substantial number of these patients are predicted to relapse before 5 years. The International Diabetes Federation criteria for optimal metabolic control after RYGB are more sensible as it encourages internationally acceptable targets to be met for glycemia, lipids, and blood pressure, without discontinuation of medication, which is unfortunately so often the case after RYGB [8]. This raises the controversy of the model of care often afforded to patients after RYGB, where many of them are prematurely and incorrectly told that they are cured of diabetes. This results in patients discontinuing their important specialist care for their chronic disease and being removed from primary care registers, thereby reducing the likelihood of appropriate long-term follow-up. The mechanisms resulting in the improved glycemia are also controversial: some proponents suggest it is all secondary to weight loss, while others suggest that additional metabolic factors may be involved [9].

Economic

Despite the high initial upfront cost of RYGB, a return on investment can be achieved within 4 years [10] due to a reduction in direct health-care costs. However, the modelling used in this type of cost assessment is questionable, and there is a dearth of controlled prospective data, especially taking into consideration the high complication rates in less experienced centers and the number of reoperations that subsequently has to be performed [11].

Functional

RYGB results in improved function status, reduced levels of back pain, and greater levels of independence. The improvement in functional ability is probably the major contributor to improved quality of life for many, but it remains unclear whether there is a threshold for weight loss that has to be exceeded before improvement can be attained. The best data would suggest that at least 20 % weight loss is needed [12], but studies confirming this threshold are lacking.

Gonadal Function and Fertility

RYGB can improve ovulatory cycles and reduce hyperandrogenism in women and may reduce maternofetal risk, although the current evidence is mainly limited to observational data. Randomized controlled data are required to allow strong recommendation on advising reproductively active women to consider RYGB prior to pregnancy.

Health Status Perceived

RYGB improves quality of life and perceived health status, with changes seen in the first year and benefit retained up to 10 years [12]. Depression, aggression, and a low self-concept can all be improved. The improvements in perceived health status and quality of life may be correlated to weight loss. However, suicide and violent death are also increased after RYGB, although the mechanisms are unclear [13]. Early reports regarding increased alcohol intake after RYGB are controversial, but may contribute [14]. It is unclear whether suicide is higher in those patients who experience significant long-term surgical complications after RYGB, because often the cause for their pain cannot be identified despite thorough investigation. Frequently, these patients are dismissed as having psychosomatic problems, resulting in them living with chronic pain and disengaging with the health-care system.

Image

Body image dysphoria is frequent in obese cohorts and often is the major drive for patients seeking RYGB. Improvement in body image satisfaction after RYGB is associated with improved quality-of-life scores, and the improvements continue following surgery. Weight regain is associated with deterioration in self-concept and body image and can be associated with symptoms of depression. In general, changes in body image are very unpredictable.

Eating disorders are also common in obese populations. RYGB can be associated with remission of eating disorders, particularly binge eating disorder. The persistence of these disorders is associated with poor outcomes, and eating behavior needs to be regularly reviewed postoperatively.

Junction of the Gastroesophagus

The combination of obesity and gastroesophageal reflux disease (GERD) has been linked with premalignant metaplasia of the gastroesophageal junction and adenocarcinoma of the esophagus. RYGB can reduce the symptoms of GERD and is associated with regression of premalignant metaplasia. The reduction in other cancers appears to be confined to females, with males not having any changes in incidence, but the mechanisms for this remain unclear [15]. The methodologies of epidemiological studies suggesting an increased risk of colorectal cancer after RYGB are being questioned, but the fact remains that no decrease in colorectal cancer has been shown after RYGB as expected initially.

Kidney Function

Obesity results in higher rates of chronic kidney disease (CKD) which is only further increased by comorbid T2DM, hypertension, or dyslipidemia. Renal parameters such as serum creatinine improve after RYGB, but this may be more to do with the reduction in lean body mass than true improvements in GFR. Attenuated urinary protein excretion after RYGB is more encouraging as it indicates a reduction in diabetic kidney damage [16]. RCTs are now needed to ascertain whether the potential benefits of RYGB outweigh the risks in those with CKD, given the greater perioperative risk associated with renal impairment.

Liver

RYGB improves the histological appearance of the liver in patients with hepatosteatosis, nonalcoholic steatohepatitis (NASH), and hepatic fibrosis, while it can lead to regression of established liver disease. However, these data are often uncontrolled and worsening in fibrosis rates after RYGB has also been reported [17].

Medication

RYGB results in a significant cost reduction in glycemic, lipid, and antihypertensive therapy, but this may be to the detriment of the patient's long-term outcomes, as many of the drugs that are stopped, such as statins, angiotensin-converting enzyme inhibitors, and metformin, have long-term mortality benefits. Additional therapies are also often needed with increased prescription of proton pump inhibitors and mineral and vitamin supplementation. These can partially offset the reductions in cost and number of tablets needed to be taken [18].

Nutritional

Deficiencies of iron, vitamin B_{12}, folate, and fat-soluble vitamins can occur after RYGB. Vomiting is not frequent after RYGB and must be considered pathological until proven otherwise. There are variable definitions and incidences of the dumping syndrome after RYGB. Symptoms 2–3 h after the meal are now being associated with postprandial hypoglycemia, although worryingly many patients may have low blood glucose without symptoms.

Other Complications

Mortality rates within 1 year due to complications of RYGB are 0.2–0.3 %, which is low in comparison with other surgical treatments [19], but high in comparison to nonsurgical treatment. Many successful weight loss drugs have been withdrawn from the market or have failed to persuade licensing authorities to allow launch, despite their demonstrating much more favorable mortality secondary to complications of treatment than surgery. Other postoperative complications include alopecia and cholelithiasis.

Purposefully Addressing the Controversies

As obesity becomes more prevalent, RYGB will be necessary for greater numbers of people. The current guidelines are aimed at a grade of obesity considered moderate to severe, but evidence is accumulating for the use of RYGB in those with BMI levels of less than 35 kg/m² [20]. This opens up the possibility to use randomized controlled trials to address the unanswered questions outlined above. It is likely that those patients with early complications of T2DM may be the cohort where the risk-to-benefit ratio is most favorable. The move to viewing RYGB as an adjuvant therapy that complements (but does not replace) existing and proven medical care may further enhance the standing of RYGB and result in a higher penetrance of this potentially helpful therapy.

References

1. Sjostrom L, Peltonen M, Jacobson P, Sjostrom CD, Karason K, Wedel H, et al. Bariatric surgery and long-term cardiovascular events. JAMA. 2012;307(1):56–65.
2. Dixon JB, Schachter LM, O'Brien PE, Jones K, Grima M, Lambert G, et al. Surgical vs conventional therapy for weight loss treatment of obstructive sleep apnea: a randomized controlled trial. JAMA. 2012;308(11):1142–9.
3. Bjorklund P, Laurenius A, Een E, Olbers T, Lonroth H, Fandriks L. Is the Roux limb a determinant for meal size after gastric bypass surgery? Obes Surg. 2010;20(10):1408–14.
4. Borg CM, le Roux CW, Ghatei MA, Bloom SR, Patel AG, Aylwin SJ. Progressive rise in gut hormone levels after Roux-en-Y gastric bypass suggests gut adaptation and explains altered satiety. Br J Surg. 2006;93(2):210–5.
5. Mathes CM, Spector AC. Food selection and taste changes in humans after Roux-en-Y gastric bypass surgery: a direct-measures approach. Physiol Behav. 2012;107(4):476–83.
6. Werling M, Olbers T, Fandriks L, Bueter M, Lonroth H, Stenlof K, et al. Increased postprandial energy expenditure may explain superior long term weight loss after Roux-en-y gastric bypass compared to vertical banded gastroplasty. PLoS One. 2013;8(4):e60280.
7. Buse JB, Caprio S, Cefalu WT, Ceriello A, Del PS, Inzucchi SE, et al. How do we define cure of diabetes? Diabetes Care. 2009;32(11):2133–5.
8. Zimmet P, Alberti KG, Rubino F, Dixon JB. IDF's view of bariatric surgery in type 2 diabetes. Lancet. 2011;378(9786):108–10.
9. Pournaras DJ, Osborne A, Hawkins SC, Vincent RP, Mahon D, Ewings P, et al. Remission of type 2 diabetes after gastric bypass and

banding: mechanisms and 2 year outcomes. Ann Surg. 2010; 252(6):966–71.

10. Cremieux PY, Ghosh A, Yang HE, Buessing M, Buchwald H, Shikora SA. Return on investment for bariatric surgery. Am J Manag Care. 2008;14(11):e5–6.

11. Maciejewski ML, Livingston EH, Smith VA, Kahwati LC, Henderson WG, Arterburn DE. Health expenditures among high-risk patients after gastric bypass and matched controls. Arch Surg. 2012;147(7):633–40.

12. Karlsson J, Taft C, Ryden A, Sjostrom L, Sullivan M. Ten-year trends in health-related quality of life after surgical and conventional treatment for severe obesity: the SOS intervention study. Int J Obes (Lond). 2007;31(8):1248–61.

13. Adams TD, Gress RE, Smith SC, Halverson RC, Simper SC, Rosamond WD, et al. Long-term mortality after gastric bypass surgery. N Engl J Med. 2007;357(8):753–61.

14. Svensson PA, Anveden A, Romeo S, Peltonen M, Ahlin S, Burza MA, et al. Alcohol consumption and alcohol problems after bariatric surgery in the swedish obese subjects study. Obesity (Silver Spring). 2013 Mar 21. doi: 10.1002/oby.20397 [Epub ahead of print].

15. Sjostrom L, Gummesson A, Sjostrom CD, Narbro K, Peltonen M, Wedel H, et al. Effects of bariatric surgery on cancer incidence in obese patients in Sweden (Swedish Obese Subjects Study): a prospective, controlled intervention trial. Lancet Oncol. 2009;10(7): 653–62.

16. Miras AD, Chuah LL, Lascaratos G, Faruq S, Mohite AA, Shah PR, et al. Bariatric surgery does not exacerbate and may be beneficial for the microvascular complications of type 2 diabetes. Diabetes Care. 2012;35(12):e81.

17. Chavez-Tapia NC, Tellez-Avila FI, Barrientos-Gutierrez T, Mendez-Sanchez N, Lizardi-Cervera J, Uribe M. Bariatric surgery for non-alcoholic steatohepatitis in obese patients. Cochrane Database Syst Rev. 2010;(1):CD007340.

18. Narbro K, Agren G, Jonsson E, Naslund I, Sjostrom L, Peltonen M. Pharmaceutical costs in obese individuals: comparison with a randomly selected population sample and long-term changes after conventional and surgical treatment: the SOS intervention study. Arch Intern Med. 2002;162(18):2061–9.

19. Flum DR, Belle SH, King WC, Wahed AS, Berk P, Chapman W, et al. Perioperative safety in the longitudinal assessment of bariatric surgery. N Engl J Med. 2009;361(5):445–54.

20. Cohen RV, Pinheiro JC, Schiavon CA, Salles JE, Wajchenberg BL, Cummings DE. Effects of gastric bypass surgery in patients with type 2 diabetes and only mild obesity. Diabetes Care. 2012;35(7): 1420–8.

Chapter 32
Weight Gain
on Glucose-Lowering Agents

Abdul Fattah Lakhdar

Introduction

Obesity increases the risk of type 2 diabetes, insulin resistance, and cardiovascular disease [1].

Ninety percent of diabetes patients are obese or overweight at diagnosis. Central obesity tends to cluster with other cardiovascular risk factors in the shape of the cardiometabolic syndrome [2]. Results of a large cross-sectional study involving a cohort of 44,042 type 2 diabetes patients from the Swedish National Diabetes Register in which 4,468 type 2 diabetes patients were studied over 6 years revealed that obese diabetes patients (37 %) had hypertension (80 %), hyperlipidemia (81 %), and microalbuminuria (29 %) where the investigators compared obese with normal and overweight-type 2 diabetes patients in relation to body mass index and cardiovascular risk factors [3].

Type 2 diabetes is a chronic condition characterized by excess micro- and macrovascular morbidity and mortality [4]. Weight reduction is fundamental for diabetes management

A.F. Lakhdar, MBChB, MSc, FRCP (Glasgow), FRCP (London)
Department of Diabetes and Endocrinology,
Barts Health NHS Trust, Whipps Cross University Hospital,
Leytonstone, London E11 1NR, UK
e-mail: abdulfattah.lakhdar@bartshealth.nhs.uk

D.W. Haslam et al. (eds.), *Controversies in Obesity*,   263
DOI 10.1007/978-1-4471-2834-2_32,
© Springer-Verlag London 2014

in overweight and obese patients with diabetes and has been shown to improve glycemic control and reduce cardiovascular risk. Hyperglycemia is a risk factor for these complications; therefore, good glycemic control is a major therapeutic target for people with type 2 diabetes [5]. The benefits of sustained glycemic control have been shown in the United Kingdom Prospective Diabetes Study (UKPDS), which found that a 0.9 % decrease in hemoglobin A1C in the intensive treatment group was associated with a 25 % reduction in microvascular complications when compared with conventional treatment.

Where lifestyle modification has failed to result in appropriate glycemic control, metformin is now universally recommended as the first-line treatment for patients with type 2 diabetes. However, treatment failure is common within 3 years, occurring in over 40 % of patients on metformin alone [6], resulting in the need for multiple oral antidiabetic agents with or without insulin. Traditional diabetes therapeutic agents including sulfonylureas, meglitinides, insulin, and thiazolidinediones often lead to undesirable weight gain, which offsets the benefit of good glycemic control [7]. Increasing weight by drugs is of particular concern as it amplifies cardiovascular risk in an already high-risk population, each 5-kg gain in weight increasing coronary heart disease risk by 30 % [7]. In the UKPDS, which established the benefit of tight glucose control on microvascular complications of type 2 diabetes patients, weight gain was significantly higher in the intensive group (mean 2.9 kg) than the conventional group ($P < 0.001$) [8]. Patients assigned to insulin had a greater weight gain (4.0 kg) than those assigned to chlorpropamide (2.6 kg) or glibenclamide (1.7 kg). In people with diabetes, weight gain is demoralizing and reduces concordance with treatment regimens [9].

Weight reduction is fundamental for diabetes management in overweight and obese patients with diabetes. It is associated with increased insulin sensitivity [10] and has the potential to lower blood pressure [11], serum total cholesterol, and triglycerides [12] and to reduce markers of inflammation, coagulation, and endothelial dysfunction [13, 14]. Consequently, weight reduction may be beneficial in reducing cardiovascular risk [15] in addition to beneficial effect on glycemic control [7]. In high-risk prediabetes individuals, weight reduction has been shown to decrease the incidence of diabetes [16].

Antidiabetic Medications with Weight Gain Potential

Insulin Secretagogues

Insulin secretagogues, such as sulfonylureas (SUs), repaglinide, and nateglinide, are effective medications in controlling hyperglycemia. SUs enhance insulin production from pancreatic beta cells through stimulation of the sulfonylurea receptors [17]. In general, SUs are known to induce weight gain; however, the amount of weight gain is variable according to the compound used and the duration of its exposure. The UKPDS [18] showed that glibenclamide and chlorpropamide caused more weight gain in comparison to diet intervention (Fig. 32.1).

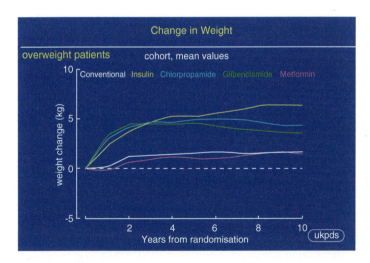

Figure. 32.1 Weight changes on glibenclamide, chlorpropamide, and insulin in comparison to diet intervention (UKPDS)

Regardless of the initial response to diet, patients on SUs gain 5-kg weight on average over a 6-year period [19], with most of this weight gain occurring during the first year [19]. The European GUIDE study is a large-scale head-to-head comparison of two once-daily administration sulfonylurea agents used in normal everyday clinical practice. In this study, 845 type 2 patients were randomized to either glimepiride or gliclazide MR in a double-blind, 27-week, parallel group design [20]. HbA1c reduction was similar in both groups (1 and 1.1 %) and body weight increased by 0.6 kg in the two groups. As monotherapy, SUs caused more weight gain than either metformin [21, 22] or repaglinide [23] and also caused more weight gain when added to pioglitazone [24] or to insulin [25]. However, the weight gain associated with SUs is similar to that caused by pioglitazone [24] and less than that caused by insulin [18].

In a randomized, parallel group, open-label, multicenter 16-week clinical trial that compared efficacy and safety of repaglinide monotherapy and nateglinide monotherapy in type 2 diabetes patients previously treated with diet and exercise [26], final HbA1c levels were lower for repaglinide monotherapy than nateglinide monotherapy (7.3 % vs. 7.9 %, respectively), $P = 0.002$. Mean weight gain at the end of the study was 1.8 kg in the repaglinide group and 0.7 kg in the nateglinide group [26].

In a head-to-head comparison over 1 year, repaglinide caused less weight gain than glyburide in pharmacotherapy-naive patients, but the difference was nonsignificant [23]. Nateglinide in combination with metformin induced more weight gain than metformin used alone after 24 weeks of treatment [27], and a published meta-analysis confirmed that patients on nateglinide gained weight in comparison to metformin [28]. Given the insulin-inducing mechanism of action of meglitinides, it is not surprising that they induce weight gain.

Insulin secretagogue-induced weight gain may be related to decreased glycosuria, increased food intake to compensate for hypoglycemia, and/or regular snacking for prevention of hypoglycemia [7]. In the UKPDS study, 27.8 % of patients treated with glibenclamide monotherapy had hypoglycemic episodes in comparison to 1.2 % in those treated with diet only [29].

Thiazolidinediones

Thiazolidinediones (TZDs) improve insulin sensitivity and promote differentiation of fat cells through their effect on peroxisome proliferator-activated receptor gamma (PPAR-γ) [30, 31]. They are antidiabetic agents that reduce insulin resistance in peripheral tissues and decrease hepatic blood glucose production. When PPAR-γ receptors are activated by a TZD, the expression of insulin-dependent glucose transporters, GLUT-4, is enhanced, followed by an upregulation of genes involved in the transport and synthesis of fatty acids [32, 33]. They act as a central regulator of adipose differentiation, promoting the production of small, more insulin-sensitive fat cells. They also act via other factors, such as increasing adiponectin and decreasing free fatty acids and TNF-α [33]. Their effect on glycemic control is more durable than metformin and SUs [34].

Weight gain has been identified as a class effect of TZD therapy [35] in several randomized, double-blind, placebo-controlled studies. The Diabetes Outcome Progression Trial (ADOPT) compared the efficacy of rosiglitazone, glyburide, and metformin in recently diagnosed patients with type 2 diabetes [34]. Patients treated with rosiglitazone gained significantly more weight than those treated with either metformin or glyburide [34]. Over 4 years, the rosiglitazone arm gained in average 2.5 kg [34]. Although their waist circumference also increased significantly, their waist-to-hip ratio did not change. The Diabetes Reduction with Rosiglitazone and Ramipril Medications (DREAM) trial [36] was conducted in a population with impaired glucose tolerance or impaired fasting glycemia. Rosiglitazone was compared with placebo over a 3-year period and reduced incident type 2 diabetes by

60 % and increased the likelihood of regression to normoglycemia [36]. Patients randomized to rosiglitazone gained an average of 3.3 kg over 36 months. Of note, compared with placebo, patients on rosiglitazone had a significant decrease in the waist-to hip ratio, with a significant increase in hip circumference, suggesting weight gain occurred peripherally as opposed to centrally [36], possibly contributing to improved insulin sensitivity. Weight gain was also observed in studied with pioglitazone. In a 23-week randomized, double-blind clinical trial, pioglitazone used as monotherapy was associated with 1.35-kg weight gain in comparison to placebo -1.87 kg ($p < 0.001$) [37, 38]. Similar effect on body weight was seen when pioglitazone was used in combination with metformin [39], SUs [40], or insulin [41]. In a 56-week randomized clinical trial, pioglitazone induced similar weight gain to glyburide, but it resulted in lower incidence of hypoglycemia and cardiac events [24]. After 104 weeks of adding pioglitazone to oral antidiabetic drugs in poorly controlled patients with type 2 diabetes, an average 3-kg weight gain was observed [42]. In one study, pioglitazone added to insulin for 24 weeks induced an average 3 kg of weight gain [43]. TZDs induced less weight gain when combined with metformin [44]. Weight gain was more prominent in patients on higher doses of TZDs and in patients with higher body mass index (BMI) at baseline.

The mechanism of weight gain with TZDs, although not totally clear, could be related to enhanced differentiation of newer fat cells through their effect on PPAR-γ receptors in the adipose tissue [30, 45]. In a randomized, double-blind, placebo-controlled trial, pioglitazone increased subcutaneous but not visceral fat over 24 weeks of intervention [46].

Insulin

Type 2 diabetes is a progressive disease characterized by a gradual decline of beta-cell function over time [47]. Not surprisingly, most type 2 diabetes patients eventually need insulin therapy for the control of hyperglycemia.

However, insulin initiation is often delayed despite deteriorating glycemic control on oral hypoglycemic drugs. In the Diabetes Attitudes, Wishes, and Needs (DAWN) study, insulin therapy was delayed until absolutely necessary [48]. Reluctance to prescribe insulin is generally for concerns of hypoglycemia and weight gain, which become a psychological barrier [49]. Insulin-associated weight gain is related to improved glycemic control and insulin dosage [7]. Weight gain is on average 2–3 kg over a 6- to 12-month period and is more limited with combination therapy than when used in monotherapy or with added metformin [50]. Some forms of insulin may cause less weight gain than others, and timing of injection and the regimen used may influence the amount gained. For example, NPH insulin, given in a single evening dose in combination with oral antidiabetic agents, induced less weight gain than four other regimens that included NPH insulin [51]. Similarly, combining bedtime NPH insulin with SUs has less impact on body weight than combining it with premeal short-acting insulin [52].

Insulin glargine and insulin detemir have a relatively delayed and prolonged absorption time and, therefore, a more predictable glucose-lowering effect compared with NPH insulin [53]. In comparison to NPH insulin, glargine induced significantly less weight gain in patients with type 1 diabetes after 16 weeks [54]. A similar observation was seen in patients with type 2 diabetes mellitus after 28 weeks [55]. However, the difference between the two insulin formulations was not seen after 52 weeks of intervention [56]. Treating to target in type 2 diabetes or 4 T [57], a 3-year open-label, multicenter trial evaluated 708 patients with suboptimal HbA1c on metformin and SU therapy. Patients were randomly assigned to receive biphasic insulin aspart twice daily, prandial insulin aspart three times daily, or basal insulin detemir once daily (twice if required). SU therapy was replaced by a second type of insulin if hyperglycemia became unacceptable during the first year of the study or subsequently if glycated hemoglobin levels were more than 6.5 %. Outcome measures were HbA1c, the proportion of patients with HbA1c of 6.5 % or less, the rate of hypoglycemia, and weight gain. Median HbA1c was similar for patients receiving biphasic (7.1 %), prandial (6.8 %), and basal (6.9 %) insulin-based regimens ($P=0.28$), and weight gain was observed in all three groups; however, the mean weight gain was higher in the prandial group than in either the biphasic group or the basal group [57]. Detemir induces less weight gain than other insulin preparations. In a large trial of >10,000 participants with type 1 and type 2 diabetes, weight did not change significantly from baseline after 14.5 weeks [58]. In a 52-week randomized, open-label, multinational trial, detemir induced less weight gain in comparison to glargine [59]. In a different study, detemir induced less weight gain compared to NPH insulin after 24 weeks [51]. It is not clear why detemir induces less weight gain than insulin comparators, although the associated frequency of hypoglycemia might be one reason. In comparison to NPH, detemir caused less hypoglycemia [60]; hence, there was reduced defensive snacking to prevent hypoglycemia [61]. Additional proposed mechanisms as potential contributors are the anabolic effects of insulin and increased lipogenesis in muscles and adipose tissues, the attenuation of insulin-evoked satiety leading to increased food intake [7], and enhanced lipogenesis due to loss of first-pass effect of subcutaneously injected insulin in contrast to endogenously secreted into portal circulation [7].

Conclusion

Weight gain may be a barrier to achieving tight glycemic control and may further aggravate the cardiovascular risk characteristic of type 2 diabetes. This is particularly problematic with insulin and insulin secretagogues. Thiazolidinediones are strong insulin sensitizers, but they generally cause significant weight gain. During weight management, their dose should be reduced but not discontinued, although newer therapeutic agents that are weight neutral or have the potential of weight reduction are generally preferred. Insulin detemir appears to reduce the risk of weight gain compared with NPH and glargine insulin. Metformin in combination therapy appears to offset to some extent the effects of weight gain of insulin and insulin secretagogues.

Editorial Comment

This chapter describes the unfortunate and damaging weight gain induced by some popular glucose-lowering agents. The fact that agents exist that attenuate weight gain, or are weight neutral, or even weight loss inducing makes the use of more primitive agents all the more troubling.

Most people with type 2 diabetes are overweight or obese; furthermore, iatrogenic weight gain is problematic with traditional glucose-lowering drugs. The use of drugs that induce dangerous, inconvenient, and demoralizing weight gain is unfortunate in an era where alternative therapies exist. Of the total costs surrounding diabetes, only 6.1 % is spent on glucose-lowering agents, whereas 86 % is spent on the consequences of using the wrong drugs – the costs of blood monitoring, hypos, hospital admissions, GP visits, etc. A small increase in direct drug costs equates to a large financial saving in overall spending.

Liraglutide, in combination with metformin, has been shown to induce weight loss of 2.6–2.9 kg for a 1.2-mg dose, and 2.8–3.4 kg for a 1.8-mg dose after 26 weeks. Liraglutide is currently being investigated at a dose of 3.0 mg in nondiabetic patients, purely as a weight loss agent, and has already been assessed against orlistat, displaying a superior weight loss of 7.2 kg compared to 4.1 kg, with 76 % of subjects, compared to 44 % losing >5 % of body weight. Exenatide demonstrates significant weight loss – up to 5.3 kg after 3 years of treatment. Albiglutide, semaglutide, and lixisenatide are novel GLP-1 mimetics currently being studied and demonstrate various degrees of weight loss.

DPP-4 inhibitors – the gliptins – are deemed weight neutral, although, like metformin, weight loss is not unexpected when it occurs.

Dapagliflozin, a recently launched renal SGLT-2 inhibitor, inhibits glucose reabsorption in the renal proximal tubule, allowing significant excretion of glucose in the urine. In trials, it induced weight loss of around 3 kg, sustained at 102 weeks compared to placebo, and primarily accounted for by reductions in total-body fat mass and in visceral and subcutaneous adipose tissue. More agents in the same class, including canagliflozin, are under development.

In the current climate of newer glucose-lowering agents being available on formulary, which are not problematic in terms of weight gain, given that diabetic subjects are almost certain to exhibit excess weight, extra consideration should be given to these "weight-friendly" compounds.

References

1. Eberhardt MS, Ogden C, Engelgau M, Cadwell B, Hedley AA, Saydah SH. Prevalence of overweight and obesity among adults with diagnosed diabetes—United States, 1988–1994 and 1999–2002. Morb Mortal Wkly Rep. 2004;53:1066–8.
2. Castro JP, El-Atar FA, McFarlane SI, Aneja A, Sowers JR. Cardiomebolic syndrome: pathophysiology and treatment. Curr Hypertens Rep. 2003;5:393–401.
3. Ridderstrale M, Gudbjornsdottir S, Eliasson B, Nilsson PM, Cederholm J, Steering Committee of the Swedish National Diabetes Register (NDR). Obesity and cardiovascular risk factors in type 2 diabetes: results from the Swedish National Diabetes Register. Intern Med. 2006;259:314–22.
4. McFarlane SI, Banarji M, Sowers JR. Insulin resistance and cardiovascular disease. Clin Endocrinol Metab. 2001;86:713–8.

5. Nathan DM, Buse JB, Davidson MB, Ferrannini E, Holman RR, Sherwin R, et al. Medical management of hyperglycaemia in type 2 diabetes: a consensus algorithm for the initiation and adjustment of therapy. Diabetes Care. 2009;32:1–11.

6. Brown JB, Conner C, Nichols GA. Secondary failure of metformin monotherapy in clinical practice. Diabetes Care. 2010;33:501–6.

7. Hermansen K, Mortensen LS. Body weight changes associated with antihyperglycaemic agents in type 2 diabetes mellitus. Drug Saf. 2007;30:1127–42.

8. Intensive blood glucose control with sulfonylureas or insulin compared with conventional treatment and the risk of complications in patients with type diabetes (UKPDS 33).UK Prospective Diabetes Study (UKPDS) Group. Lancet. 1998;352(9131):837–53.

9. Guisasola FA, Povedano ST, Krishnarajah G, Lyu R, Mavros P, Yin D. Hypoglycaemic symptoms, treatment satisfaction, adherence and their associations with glycaemic goal in patients with type 2 diabetes mellitus: findings from the Real-Life Effectiveness and Care Patterns of Diabetes Management (RECAP-DM) Study. Diabetes Obes Metab. 2008;10:S25–32.

10. Hamdy O, Ledbury S, Mullooly C, Jarema C, Porter S, Ovalle K, et al. Lifestyle modification improves endothelial function in obese subjects with the insulin resistance syndrome. Diabetes Care. 2003;26(7):2119–25.

11. Mertens IL, Van Gaal LF. Overweight, obesity, and blood pressure: the effects of modest weight reduction. Obes Res. 2000;8(3):270–8.

12. Metz JA, Stern JS, Kris-Etherton P, Reusser ME, Morris CD, Hatton DC, et al. A randomized trial of improved weight loss with a prepared meal plan in overweight and obese patients: impact on cardiovascular risk reduction. Arch Intern Med. 2000;160(14):2150–8.

13. Monzillo LU, Hamdy O, Horton ES, Ledbury S, Mullooly C, Jarema C, et al. Effect of lifestyle modification on adipokine levels in obese subjects with insulin resistance. Obes Res. 2003;11(9):1048–54.

14. Ziccardi P, Nappo F, Giugliano G, Esposito K, Marfella R, Cioffi M, et al. Reduction of inflammatory cytokine concentrations and improvement of endothelial functions in obese women after weight loss over one year. Circulation. 2002;105(7):804–9.

15. Williams KV, Kelley DE. Metabolic consequences of weight loss on glucose metabolism and insulin action in type 2 diabetes. Diabetes Obes Metab. 2000;2(3):121–9.

16. Muniyappa R, El-Atat F, Aneja A, McFarlane SI. The diabetes prevention program. Curr Diab Rep. 2003;3:221–2.

17. Lebovitz HE. Oral hypoglycaemic agents. Prim Care. 1988;15:353–69.

18. Intensive blood-glucose control with sulphonylurea or insulin compared with conventional treatment and risk of complications in patients with type 2 diabetes (UKPDS 33). UK Prospective Diabetes Study (UKPDS) Group. Lancet. 1998; 352(9131):837–53.

19. United Kingdom Prospective Diabetes Study 24: a 6-year, randomized, controlled trial comparing sulfonylurea, insulin, and metformin therapy in patients with newly diagnosed type 2 diabetes that could not be controlled with diet therapy. United Kingdom Prospective Diabetes Study Group. Ann Intern Med. 1998;128(3):165–75.

20. Shernthaner G, Grimaldi A, Di Mario U, Drzewoski J, Kempler P, Kvapil M, et al. GUIDE study: double-blind comparison of once-daily gliclazide MR and glimepiride in type 2 diabetic patients. Eur J Clin Invest. 2004;34:535–42.

21. Campbell IW, Menzies DG, Chalmers J, McBain AM, Brown IR. One year comparative trial of metformin and glipizide in type 2 diabetes mellitus. Diabete Metab. 1994;20(4):394–400.

22. Hermann LS, Schersten B, Bitzen PO, Kjellström T, Lindgärde F, Melander A. Therapeutic comparison of metformin and sulfonylurea, alone and in various combinations. A double-blind controlled study. Diabetes Care. 1994;17(10):1100–9.

23. Marbury T, Huang WC, Strange P, Lebovitz H. Repaglinide versus glyburide: a one-year comparison trial. Diabetes Res Clin Pract. 1999;43(3):155–66.

24. Jain R, Osei K, Kupfer S, Perez AT, Zhang J. Long-term safety of pioglitazone versus glyburide in patients with recently diagnosed type 2 diabetes mellitus. Pharmacotherapy. 2006;26(10):1388–95.

25. Lewitt MS, Yu VK, Rennie GC, Carter JN, Marel GM, Yue DK, et al. Effects of combined insulin-sulfonylurea therapy in type II patients. Diabetes Care. 1989;12(6):379–83.

26. Rosenstock J, Hassman DR, Madder RD, Brazinsky SA, Farrell J, Khutoryansky N, et al. Repaglinide versus nateglinide monotherapy: a randomized multicenter study. Diabetes Care. 2004;27:1265–70.

27. Marre M, Van Gaal L, Usadel KH, Ball M, Whatmough I, Guitard C. Nateglinide improves glycaemic control when added to metformin monotherapy: results of a randomized trial with type 2 diabetes patients. Diabetes Obes Metab. 2002;4(3):177–86.

28. Black C, Donnelly P, McIntyre L, Royle PL, Shepherd JP, Thomas S. Meglitinide analogues for type 2 diabetes mellitus. Cochrane Database Syst Rev 2007;(2):CD004654.

29. United Kingdom Prospective Diabetes Study (UKPDS). 13: relative efficacy of randomly allocated diet, sulphonylurea, insulin, or metformin in patients with newly diagnosed non-insulin-dependent diabetes followed for three years. BMJ. 1995;310(6972):83–8.

30. Braissant O, Foufelle F, Scotto C, Dauça M, Wahli W. Differential expression of peroxisome proliferator-activated receptors (PPARs): tissue distribution of PPAR-alpha, -beta, and -gamma in the adult rat. Endocrinology. 1996;137(1):354–66. Gosset P, Charbonnier AS, Delerive P, Fontaine J, Staels B, Pestel J, et al. Peroxisome proliferator-activated receptor gamma activators affect the maturation of human monocyte-derived dendritic cells. Eur J Immunol. 2001;31(10):2857–65.

31. Goldstein BJ, Scalia R. Adiponectin: a novel adipokine linking adipocytes and vascular function. J Clin Endocrinol Metab. 2004; 89(6):2563–8.

32. Phillips SA, Ciaraldi TP, Kong AP, Bandukwala R, Aroda V, Carter L, et al. Modulation of circulating and adipose tissue adiponectin levels by antidiabetic therapy. Diabetes. 2003;52(3):667–74.

33. Spiegelman BM. PPAR-gamma: adipogenic regulator and thiazolidinedione receptor. Diabetes. 1998;47:1265–70.

34. Viberti G, Kahn SE, Greene DA, Herman WH, Zinman B, Holman RR, et al. A diabetes outcome progression trial (ADOPT): an international multicenter study of the comparative efficacy of rosiglitazone, glyburide, and metformin in recently diagnosed type 2 diabetes. Diabetes Care. 2002;25(10):1737–43.

35. Wilding J. Thiazolidinediones, insulin resistance and obesity: finding a balance. Int J Clin Pract. 2006;60:1272–80.

36. DREAM (Diabetes REduction Assessment with ramipril and rosiglitazone Medication) Trial Investigators, Gerstein HC, Yusuf S, Bosch J, Pogue J, Sheridan P, Dinccag N, et al. Effect of rosiglitazone on the frequency of diabetes in patients with impaired glucose tolerance or impaired fasting glucose: a randomised controlled trial. Lancet. 2006;368:1096–105.

37. Aronoff S, Rosenblatt S, Braithwaite S, Egan JW, Mathisen AL, Schneider RL. Pioglitazone hydrochloride monotherapy improves glycemic control in the treatment of patients with type 2 diabetes: a 6-month randomized placebo-controlled dose–response study. The Pioglitazone 001 Study Group. Diabetes Care. 2000;23(11):1605–11.

38. Rosenblatt S, Miskin B, Glazer NB, Prince MJ, Robertson KE. Pioglitazone 026 Study Group. The impact of pioglitazone on glycemic control and atherogenic dyslipidaemia in patients with type 2 diabetes mellitus. Coron Artery Dis. 2001;12(5):413–23.

39. Einhorn D, Rendell M, Rosenzweig J, Egan JW, Mathisen AL, Schneider RL. Pioglitazone hydrochloride in combination with metformin in the treatment of type 2 diabetes mellitus: a randomized, placebo-controlled study. The Pioglitazone 027 Study Group. Clin Ther. 2000;22(12):1395–409.

40. Kipnes MS, Krosnick A, Rendell MS, Egan JW, Mathisen AL, Schneider RL. Pioglitazone hydrochloride in combination with sulfonylurea therapy improves glycemic control in patients with type 2 diabetes mellitus: a randomized, placebo-controlled study. Am J Med. 2001;111(1):10–7.

41. Davidson JA, Perez A, Zhang J. Addition of pioglitazone to stable insulin therapy in patients with poorly controlled type 2 diabetes: results of a double-blind, multicentre, randomized study. Diabetes Obes Metab. 2006;8(2):164–74.

42. Charbonnel B, Schernthaner G, Brunetti P, Matthews DR, Urquhart R, Tan MH, et al. Long-term efficacy and tolerability of add-on

pioglitazone therapy to failing monotherapy compared with addition of gliclazide or metformin in patients with type 2 diabetes. Diabetologia. 2005;48(6):1093–104.

43. Davidson J, Vexiau P, Cucinotta D, Vaz J, Kawamori R. Biphasic insulin aspart 30: literature review of adverse events associated with treatment. Clin Ther. 2005;27(Suppl B):S75–88.

44. Fonseca V, Rosenstock J, Patwardhan R, Salzman A. Effect of metformin and rosiglitazone combination therapy in patients with type 2 diabetes mellitus: a randomized controlled trial. JAMA. 2000;283(13):1695–702.

45. Braissant O, Foufelle F, Scotto C, Dauça M, Wahli W. Differential expression of peroxisome proliferator-activated receptors (PPARs): tissue distribution of PPAR-alpha, -beta, and -gamma in the adult rat. Endocrinology. 1996;137(1):354–66.

46. Smith SR, De Jonge L, Volaufova J, Li Y, Xie H, Bray GA. Effect of pioglitazone on body composition and energy expenditure: a randomized controlled trial. Metabolism. 2005;54(1):24–32.

47. UK prospective Diabetes Study 16. Overview of 6 years therapy of type II diabetes: U.K. Prospective Diabetes Study Group. Diabetes. 1995; 44:1249–58.

48. Peyrot M, Rubin RR, Lauritzen T, Skovlund SE, Snoek FJ, Matthews DR, et al. Resistance to insulin therapy among patients and providers: results of the cross-national Diabetes Attitudes, Wishes, and Needs (DAWN) study. Diabetes Care. 2005;28:2673–9.

49. Carver C. Insulin treatment and the problem of weight gain in type 2 diabetes. Diabetes Educ. 2006;32:910–7.

50. Goodswaard AN, Furlong NJ, Rutten GE, Stolk RP, Valk GD. Insulin monotherapy versus combination of insulin with oral hypoglycaemic agents in patients with type 2 diabetes mellitus. Cochrane Database Syst Rev. 2004;4, CD003418.

51. Yki-Jarvinen H, Kauppila M, Kujansuu E, Lahti J, Marjanen T, Niskanen L, et al. Comparison of insulin regimens in patients with non-insulin-dependent diabetes mellitus. N Engl J Med. 1992; 327(20):1426–33.

52. Clauson P, Karlander S, Steen L, Efendic S. Daytime glibenclamide and bedtime NPH insulin compared to intensive insulin treatment in secondary sulphonylurea failure: a 1-year follow-up. Diabet Med. 1996;13(5):471–7.

53. Meneghini L. Why and how to use insulin therapy earlier in the management of type 2 diabetes. South Med J. 2007;100:164–74.

54. Raskin P, Klaff L, Bergenstal R, Hallé JP, Donley D, Mecca T. A 16-week comparison of the novel insulin analog insulin glargine (HOE 901) and NPH human insulin used with insulin lispro in patients with type 1 diabetes. Diabetes Care. 2000;23(11):1666–71.

55. Rosenstock J, Schwartz SL, Clark Jr CM, Park GD, Donley DW, Edwards MB. Basal insulin therapy in type 2 diabetes: 28-week

comparison of insulin glargine (HOE 901) and NPH insulin. Diabetes Care. 2001;24(4):631–6.

56. Yki-Jarvinen H, Dressler A, Ziemen M. Less nocturnal hypoglyce-mia and better post-dinner glucose control with bedtime insulin glargine compared with bedtime NPH insulin during insulin combi-nation therapy in type 2 diabetes. HOE 901/3002 Study Group. Diabetes Care. 2000;23(8):1130–6.

57. Holman RR, Andrew J, Farmer AJ, Melanie J, Davies MJ, Keenan JF, et al. Three-year efficacy of complex insulin regimens in type 2 dia-betes. N Engl J Med. 2009;361:1736–47.

58. Meneghini LF, Rosenberg KH, Koenen C, Merilainen MJ, Lüddeke HJ. Insulin detemir improves glycaemic control with less hypogly-caemia and no weight gain in patients with type 2 diabetes who were insulin naive or treated with NPH or insulin glargine: clinical prac-tice experience from a German subgroup of the PREDICTIVE study. Diabetes Obes Metab. 2007;9(3):418–27.

59. Rosenstock J, Davies M, Home P, Larsen J, Koenen C, Schernthaner G. Randomised, 52-week, treat-to-target trial comparing insulin detemir with insulin glargine when administered as add-on to glucose-lowering drugs in insulin-naive people with type 2 diabetes. Diabetologia. 2008;51(3):408–16.

60. Heller S. Weight gain during insulin therapy in patients with type 2 diabetes mellitus. Diabetes Res Clin Pract. 2004;65 Suppl 1:S23–7.

61. Kolendorf K, Ross GP, Pavlic-Renar I, Perriello G, Philotheou A, Jendle J, et al. Insulin detemir lowers the risk of hypoglycaemia and provides more consistent plasma glucose levels compared with NPH insulin in type 1 diabetes. Diabet Med. 2006;23(7):729–35.

Chapter 33
Tipping the Scales of Truth: Why the Energy Balance Equation Is a Dangerous Lie

Damian Edwards

Calories in, calories out. Energy in, energy out. Simple, isn't it? Apparently, the more we eat and the less we exercise, the more weight we gain. So if we want to get rid of some weight, we have two choices – eat less or exercise more.

For too long now we have accepted the Energy Balance Equation as the principal tool with which to tackle obesity. We have focused our efforts firmly upon the idea that "A person needs to be in 'energy balance' to maintain a healthy weight – that is, their energy intake (from food) should not exceed the energy expended through everyday activities and exercise" [1].

Blindly, we sold the Energy Balance Equation to obese clients and naively assumed that it was all we needed to encourage smaller portions and more activity. Arrogantly, we paraded this equation as a fact so obvious that if only people could follow its inescapable logic, then they would be slim, healthy, and happy.

In truth, only one fact is glaringly obvious – that in the "Fight against Fat," our insistence on the Energy Equation has failed. Focusing on the math, we have missed the humanity. Despite its "inescapable logic," the Energy Equation has

D. Edwards, BA Hons
Department of Behavioural Interventions,
National Obesity Forum, Unit 1.03, Enterprise
House, 1/2 Hatfields, London, SE1 9PG, UK
e-mail: info@hdm-medical.com

D.W. Haslam et al. (eds.), *Controversies in Obesity*,
DOI 10.1007/978-1-4471-2834-2_33,
© Springer-Verlag London 2014

become *a dangerous lie* – oversimplified, inadequate, and misleading, addressing none of the important cognitive and behavioral questions:

- WHY do we overeat?
- WHAT does food mean to us?
- HOW do we change our relationship with food?

Cogent, academic articles have argued that "Increasing obesity in the face of decreasing food intake can only be explained if levels of energy expenditure have declined faster than energy intake, thus leading to an overconsumption of energy relative to a greatly reduced requirement" [2].

Can obesity really be reduced to a mathematical formula? Can increasing obesity "*only be explained*" in terms of energy and/or metabolism? The same author states, "Escalating rates of obesity are occurring in a relatively constant gene pool and hence against a constant metabolic background" [2].

Civilized societies are getting heavier, and obesity is an epidemic that is spreading across all levels of society [3]. Not just the disadvantaged, also financially fortunate individuals are failing, trapped in unhealthy snacking patterns, yo-yo diets or the latest destructive fad, despite access to the foods and facilities for a healthier lifestyle.

So why are we getting fatter not fitter? Why are we witness to an obesity epidemic in the UK that "threatens to bankrupt the healthcare system" [4] because it is "out of control, and none of the measures being undertaken show signs of halting the problem, let alone reversing the trend" [4].

The fault is that we have promoted a lie that continues to mislead both professionals and public alike. Obsessed with energy balance, we have overlooked the real issues around behavior, psychology, emotion, and self-esteem. *We* have focused on food and asked our patients to do the same, reducing the complex psychosocial conundrum of hyperphagic behavior to a childish calorie-counting exercise. It is an insult to our patients and an embarrassment to the medical profession.

The deeper human truth is just as clear but a damn sight less convenient: *In the fight against obesity, at an individual or societal level, the solution has less to do with WHAT we eat and more to do with what we THINK and FEEL when we eat.*

We do not overeat because we are hungry – we overeat because we are sad, lonely, frustrated, unfulfilled, angry, and hurt. We reach for food because we have been taught to believe that it will comfort us. Yet the proof is in the pudding – we are getting fatter and not happier. Depression, like obesity, is also on the increase. Why? The answer is this: *We can never get enough of what we don't really want – and food is not really what we want.*

When we reach for food in an attempt to satisfy deep human emotional needs, we will always fail. If we eat out of loneliness, food is no kind of companion. If our job is stressful or we are unhappy in a relationship, things will be just the same after that burger. Our lives are not less miserable when we overeat. Emotional eating solves no problems but causes many.

One Cochrane Review concluded that people who are overweight or obese benefit from psychological interventions, particularly behavioral and cognitive-behavioral strategies [5].

Yet what are we still teaching the people we are supposedly helping? *Calories in, calories out. Simple! Just eat less and exercise more – Next!*

Remember the old joke about the guy who visits the doctor and, when asked what is wrong, he raises his arm high and explains: "Doctor, it hurts when I do this." The doctor looks at him drily and replies: "Then don't do it." Our insistence on the glib, uncomplicated retort of "Eat less and exercise more" is just as unhelpful. The Energy Equation is at best naive and, at its worst, it is the sticking plaster of jaded, overworked staff under pressure of ever shorter appointments, pushed to reduce human behavior to "quick and easy" answers that simply never work.

We need to tackle obesity at its root – applying principles from behavioral and cognitive behavioral therapies to understand *why* we eat and *how* we can change. We ought to be addressing the psychology that underpins overeating. This can be achieved without becoming bogged down in analysis, simply by teaching obese patients strategies for stress management and improving self-esteem. Fundamentally, we need to teach *better beliefs about food.*

At the same time, we need to address the behavioral "nudges" that trigger unhealthy levels of eating. In the UK, for example, we could lobby McDonalds for ONE simple change that would affect a nation – to ask: "Would you like *fruit* with that?' adding an apple or orange to their latest tray load.

More than anything, though, we need to stop lying to people and pretending that tackling obesity is simply an Energy Equation, because it hurts our patients and our profession when we do that *– so let's not do it.*

References

1. National Institute for Health and Clinical Excellence (NICE), NICE Clinical Guideline CG43. Obesity: guidance on the prevention, identification, assessment and management of overweight and obesity in adults and children (Dec 2006, review Dec 2011) Recommendations for the public 1.1.1 p 13. Available from: http://guidance.nice.org.uk/CG43.
2. Prentice AM, Jebb SA. Obesity in Britain: gluttony or sloth? BMJ. 1995;311(7002):437–9. Available from: http://www.ncbi.nlm.nih.gov/pmc/articles/PMC2550498/.
3. McAllister EJ, Dhurandhar NV, Keith SW, Aronne LJ, Barger J, Baskin M, et al. Ten putative contributors to the obesity epidemic. Crit Rev Food Sci Nutr. 2009;49:868–913.
4. Haslam D, Sattar N, Lean M. ABC of obesity. Obesity – time to wake up. BMJ. 2006;333:640–2.
5. Shaw KA, O'Rourke P, Del Mar C, Kenardy J. Psychological interventions for overweight or obesity. Cochrane Database Syst Rev. 2005;3:CD003818.

Chapter 34
OTC Slimming Aids

Terry Maguire

Introduction

Over-the-counter (OTC) slimming aids are claimed to act by either one or all of the following mechanisms:

1. Increase satiety
2. Decrease absorption
3. Increase fat oxidation, increase metabolic rate, or reduce lipogenesis

Most products are unlicensed; therefore, health care professionals know little about them. In a UK survey of 75 community pharmacies, it was found that 72 % of pharmacies sold one or more of these products, yet pharmacy staff received no training in their use [1]. In another survey of 460 pharmacy customers, 20 % said that they had tried an OTC weight-loss product. Some 60 % thought that an assessment of weight and height should be taken before supply of these products is made [2].

T. Maguire, BSc, PhD, FPSNI
The School of Pharmacy, The Queen's University of Belfast,
C/O 3, Beechmount Avenue, Belfast,
Antrim BT12 7NA, Northern Ireland, UK
e-mail: t.maguire@qub.ac.uk

D.W. Haslam et al. (eds.), *Controversies in Obesity*,
DOI 10.1007/978-1-4471-2834-2_34,
© Springer-Verlag London 2014

OTC slimming aids are generally formulated to look like a medicine – a capsule, a tablet, or a patch, giving the impression of a medically effective product. They are priced to be expensive and, therefore, desirable. Placement of products is mostly in pharmacies and other health outlets. For this reason, pharmacists particularly must consider the implications of stocking and selling such products [3]. Manufacturers are creative in overcoming restrictions on making medical claims. This is often done using personal testimonies used to convince others of the product's efficacy. However, some products use a loophole within European medicine regulations and are registering their products as "a medical device."

OTC Diet Aid Products

With the exception of Alli, which contains the licensed drug orlistat and which is available OTC in the USA and Europe and for which there is good evidence of safety and efficacy, there is little evidence that other OTC slimming aids work. An Zassessment of the current published evidence for the efficacy and safety of the ingredients of popular OTC slimming products is given in a number of review articles published elsewhere [4–7].

Sympathomimetic Amines

Ephedra sinica, phenylpropanolamine, Ma Huang (ephedra), and ephedrine were widely used in OTC slimming aids. Ephedrine and caffeine are effective in reducing body weight. The most rigorous review [7–9] concluded that *E. sinica* and ephedrine promote a modest short-term weight loss of about 0.9 kg/month greater than placebo. However, efficacy was associated with a threefold increase in side effects that included psychiatric events, gastrointestinal events, heart palpitations, and a dose-related increase in blood pressure. The FDA banned these products for this purpose in 2000.

Chitosan

Chitosan is a cationic polysaccharide and is derived from the shells of mainly crabs and shrimp. It has a highly adsorptive surface and for this reason is promoted as a "fat blocker." Chitosan can reduce body weight in animals; a small number of studies in humans support this, but most suffer from poor methodology. The evidence indicates that there is considerable doubt that chitosan is effective [5].

Hoodia Gordonii

Claimed to work as an appetite suppressant, manufacturers of products containing Hoodia claim it to be the first truly effective weight management product. Hoodia is derived from the cactus *Hoodia gordonii,* which grows in the Kalahari Desert. An active ingredient, P57, has been isolated, but studies on this have yet to be published.

Chromium Picolinate

Chromium is involved in carbohydrate and fat metabolism. Since chromium can enhance insulin sensitivity, decrease circulating insulin levels, and improve glucose tolerance, it has been theorized that it could increase satiety, improve body composition (ratio of lean to fat tissue), increase basal metabolic rate, and reduce body weight. There currently is no evidence to support this.

L-Carnitine and Acetyl-L-Carnitine

L-Carnitine is a cofactor in cellular fat oxidation, and in obesity fat oxidation is reduced due to a reduction in L-carnitine enzyme-related activity. For this theoretical reason, L-carnitine is promoted as a "fat burner." There is little if any evidence to support its efficacy in obese or overweight humans [4].

Green Tea

Green tea contains catechin polyphenols, which have been shown to inhibit COMT, the enzyme responsible for the degradation of noradrenaline. Since noradrenaline has an important role in the control of thermogenesis, basal metabolic rate, and fat metabolism, it has been theorized that consumption of green tea might contribute to weight loss. Work in rats has demonstrated weight loss, but this is restored once supplementation is stopped. Tea catechin has been shown to cause appetite loss, which might be the route by which the weight loss is affected.

Conjugated Linoleic Acid

Studies in rodents have demonstrated a reduction in body fat and body weight when animals were treated with CLA supplements. For this reason, conjugated linoleic acid (CLA) supplements have been promoted OTC as a weight-loss aid. However, there is little evidence that CLA supplements reduce body weight or body fat in humans. More worryingly, studies in rodents have shown that supplementation is associated with liver hypertrophy and insulin resistance, and this must be of concern to anyone wishing to use CLA supplements. Notwithstanding this, no human trials to date have demonstrated these adverse events even in higher than normal doses [4].

Hydroxycitric Acid

Hydroxycitric acid is obtained from extracts of *Garcinia cambogia* and has been shown to inhibit the citrate cleavage enzyme and suppress de novo fatty acid synthesis and food intake. In this way, it is theorized that it decreases body weight gain.

Whereas a number of studies in humans support the efficacy of HCA in weight loss, all studies suffer from significant methodological deficiencies that question the relevance of the findings [6].

Non-starch Polysaccharides (Fiber)

Based on the F-Plan diet theme, fiber-based products increase satiety and so reduce energy intake. Where this has been shown to happen, for example, in the context of the F-Plan diet, the amount of fiber needed to support and maintain weight loss is larger than the amount normally provided from fiber supplements, and there exists no evidence that these supplements can induce significant weight loss in the long term [4].

Lecithin

Lecithin is a phospholipid found in egg yolks, liver, peanuts, and soya beans. Lecithin is thought to prevent the deposition of fat in fat cells. A well-conducted Swedish study looking at the effect of lecithin supplementation and its effect on weight did not show any significant benefits in weight loss.

Guarana and Yerba Mate

Yerba mate (*Ilex paraguariensis*) is an evergreen tree that is native to South America. It is often combined in OTC weight loss preparation with guarana (*Paullinia cupana*).

Both these plants are sources of stimulant chemical agents – caffeine and xanthine, respectively. There is some evidence that extracts from these plants that are very high in caffeine have been able to prolong gastric emptying time. However, there is little evidence that, as stimulants, they are effective in raising the body's basal metabolic rate to such a degree as to cause weight loss [3].

Hydroxymethylbutyrate

Hydroxymethylbutyrate (HMB) is a metabolite of leucine that has been shown to have anti-catabolic action through inhibiting protein breakdown. Products containing HMB are primarily targeted at body builders who wish to change body composition and improve muscle mass. There is some evidence to support this outcome, but the few trials that are published have methodological problems; therefore, more studies are required.

Pyruvate

Pyruvate is created in the body through glycolysis. Supplementation with pyruvate seems to enhance exercise performance and improve measures of body composition. There exist two randomized controlled trials involving patients with BMI of 25 or greater, but neither showed any greater effect on weight compare to placebo, so the conclusion is that pyruvate as an aid to body-composition changes and weight loss is weak.

References

1. Andronicou A, Maxwell S, Hackett A, Richards J, Krska J. Availability of over the counter weight loss products from pharmacies. Int J Pharm Pract. 2007;15(Suppl):A13–4.
2. Krska J. Pharmacy staff should be proactive when selling OTC weight loss products. Pharm J. 2008;281:189.
3. Maguire T. We are what we sell. Pharm J. 2008;281:96.
4. Boon G, Lockwood B. Neutraceuticals. Pharm J. 2008;276:15–7.
5. Mason P. OTC weight control products. Pharm J. 2002;269:103–5.
6. Pittler M, Ernst E. Dietary supplements for body weight reduction: a systematic review. Am J Clin Nutr. 2004;79:529–36.
7. Hulisz D, Lindberg K. The skinny on weight loss supplements: fact or fantasy? Available from: http://www.medscape.org/viewarticle/574182_5.
8. Shekelle P, Hardy M, Morton S, Maglione M, Mojica WA, Suttorp MJ, et al. Efficacy and safety of ephedra and ephedrine for weight loss and athletic performance. JAMA. 2003;289:1537–45.
9. Dixon JB. Weight loss medications – where do they fit in? Aust Fam Physician. 2006;35:576–9.

Chapter 35
Overcoming Sloth

Fred Turok

The Epidemic

The physical inactivity pandemic is now a public health problem on the same scale as smoking, poor nutrition, and alcohol use and therefore needs a similarly robust approach.

The time to debate is over; the time to act is now.

The cost of physical inactivity in England alone has been estimated at £8.2 billion a year, and the role that physical activity can play in the prevention and management of chronic disease is well understood. Physical inactivity is the fourth leading risk factor for global mortality (6 % of deaths nationally). Conversely, physical activity reduces the risk of major noncommunicable disease, including coronary heart disease (CHD), hypertension, type 2 diabetes, and some cancers by up to 50 %, and also improves mental well-being and general quality of life. Despite these stark statistics, which point at the dangers of our currently sedentary lifestyles, levels of physical activity are inexcusably poor.

F. Turok
Department of Health,
Responsibility Deal Physical Activity Network,
77-79 New Oxford Street 3rd Floor Castlewood House,
London, WC1A 1DG, UK
e-mail: fred@ukactive.org.uk

D.W. Haslam et al. (eds.), *Controversies in Obesity*,
DOI 10.1007/978-1-4471-2834-2_35,
© Springer-Verlag London 2014

Based on recent research in England [1], only 39 % of men and 29 % of women aged 16 and over met the Chief Medical Officer's (CMO) minimum recommendations for physical activity in adults, and the percentages of both men and women who met the recommendations generally decreased with age. When based on accelerometer reporting, these percentages fell to only 6 % of men and 4 % of women. Even on the self-reported measure, 27 million people in England alone are not sufficiently active to benefit their health.

The associated cost of this inactivity is becoming burdensome on the National Health Service and will continue to do so as the population gets fatter and sicker due to sedentary behavior. On a simple scale, an inactive person spends 38 % more days in hospital than an active person and has 5.5 % more family physician visits, 13 % more specialist services, and 12 % more nurse visits than an active individual. At a time when health services globally are under severe economic pressure, these statistics are unacceptable and the focus must shift to prevention of obesity.

The Response

Action is required on a wide and impactful scale to reverse this trend before it cripples the country, leading to a "charged for NHS" and devastating health services worldwide. There is no simple answer, but what is evident is that people will not behave rationally even when faced with the facts.

There is no single answer either – flexibility is required to understand that what might engage a previously active person to become more active will differ greatly to someone who has never undertaken any exercise. A pragmatic, robust approach, using all of the resources that can realistically be afforded, is needed, meaning that strategies must be developed, bringing together all stakeholders from business, community sports participation, volunteering, education, employment, the medical community, and the digital community. Such an approach may mean working with organizations that perhaps are not traditionally associated with healthy living, and this may upset some, but the situation is too grave and too pressing to attempt to please all. Policy areas such as schools, local communities, workplaces, the Olympic legacy, and sports participation all require clearly articulated strategies; for instance, 9.8 % of children enter primary school as obese, yet twice as many (18.7 %) leave primary school as obese, therefore clearly articulating the need for a strategy in this area.

However, this chapter focuses on two issues: getting the inactive active and using the capacity within big business.

Behavior Change: Physical Activity Counselling

There are distinct groups within those that do not engage in regular physical activity – this includes those that are lapsed exercisers and those long-term inactive who have never been fully engaged. Barriers, perceived or real, to participating in physical activity need to be understood and explored before behavior can be altered sustainably. Recognizing this, the UK Department of Health commissioned the development, piloting, and evaluation of "Let's Get Moving," a physical activity behavioral intervention based on motivational interviewing. This "nudge" approach has proved remarkably successful in several programs. A pilot undertaken in Essex, England, in 2011 showed that with a user base of 504 people engaged in the program, a total 164 million steps were taken, accounting to 48,000 active hours, 11.2 million kcal, and 69,000 miles walked. For previously inactive people in danger of developing chronic diseases related to their lifestyle choices, this was a significant outcome that showed the scale of impact that can be achieved by a robust approach to delivering public health interventions. There are numerous case studies, research articles, journal entries, and examples supporting the clear message that a simple discussion with a trained exercise professional can increase activity levels in an individual who has never previously engaged in physical activity. This is a low-cost, low-intensity but high-yield intervention that should be made widely available within the UK and beyond; in other words, every GP surgery should have an exercise professional capable of delivering such an intervention.

Pragmatism: Powerful Brands and Responsible Employers

While the "Let's Get Moving" approach is an effective tool to combat inactivity among those most at need within local communities, it cannot be relied upon alone. Realistically, the scale of the problem is such that ways must be found of reaching the most amount of people in the most effective manner.

The role of business should not be overlooked – businesses reach millions of people through their brands and products every day, and they employ millions of people who sit at their desks all day every day. Between the consumers and staff that engage with business on a daily basis, it is clear that these organizations have a responsibility and a duty to act as a vehicle to promote well-being and, in particular, physical activity.

The Department of Health in the UK is setting examples: In 2010 it launched the Responsibility Deal, which seeks to find a societal response to the societal epidemic of unhealthy lifestyles. The Physical Activity Network of the Deal aims to create partnerships and pledges between business and physical activity providers in a bid to increase levels of physical activity across the country. Organizations signing up to the Responsibility Deal commit to taking action voluntarily to improve public health through their responsibilities as employers as well as through their consumer propositions and their community activities.

The result is that more than 220 organizations have already signed up and are delivering projects to increase the physical activity levels of their consumers and staff. There are, of course, criticisms and questions about to this approach.

Are all these organizations doing this purely out of altruistic motives? Definitely not.

Could some of the products on offer from these organizations be classed as unhealthy? Undeniably.

Is it palatable to have these organizations take credit for doing something positive when they make money from unhealthy products? Potentially not.

Should we be legislating instead? Maybe.

A final question: Given the urgency of the situation and the scale of the epidemic that worsens every day, do we have a choice?

Absolutely not.

Reference

1. Health and Social Care Information Centre. Health Survey for England – 2008. Published Dec 17, 2009. Available from: http://www. hscic.gov.uk/pubs/hse08physicalactivity.

Index

D.W. Haslam et al. (eds.), *Controversies in Obesity*,
DOI 10.1007/978-1-4471-2834-2,
© Springer-Verlag London 2014

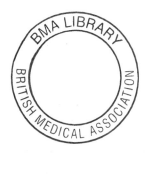

Printed by Printforce, the Netherlands